TRAIN LIKE A BODYBUILDER

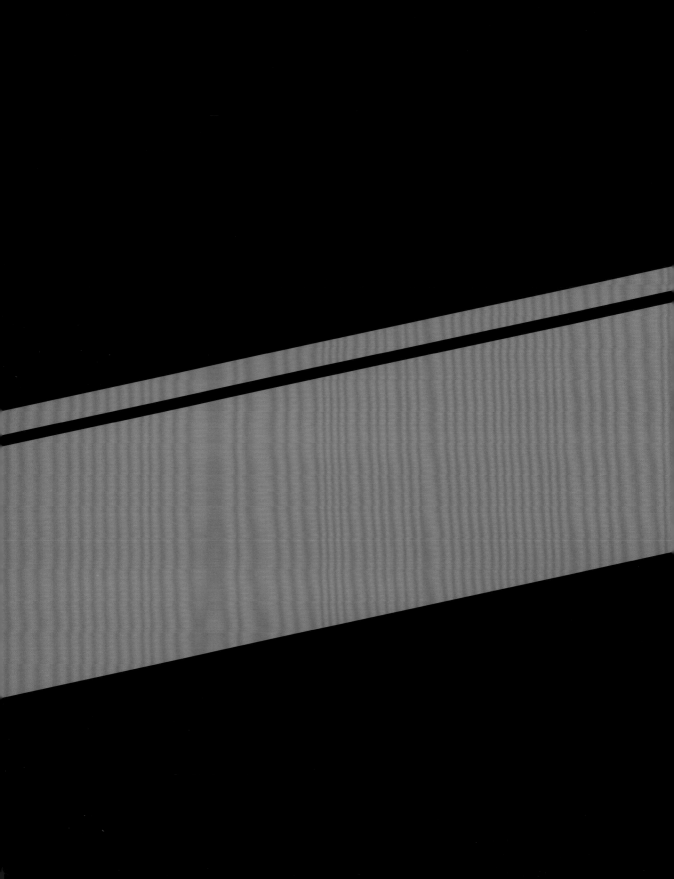

ERIN STERN

TRAIN LIKE A BODYBUILDER

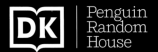

Publisher Mike Sanders
Senior Editor Brook Farling
Senior Designer Becky Batchelor
Art Director William Thomas
Photographer Elese Bales
Proofreader Lisa Starnes
Indexer Celia McCoy

First American Edition, 2019
Published in the United States by DK Publishing
6081 E. 82nd Street, Indianapolis, Indiana 46250

A catalog record for this book
is available from the Library of Congress.
ISBN: 978-1-4654-8374-4
Library of Congress Catalog Number: 2018960709

DK books are available at special discounts when purchased in bulk for sales
promotions, premiums, fundraising, or educational use. For details, contact: DK
Publishing Special Markets, 1450 Broadway, Suite 801, New York, NY 10018
SpecialSales@dk.com

Printed and bound in China

All images © Dorling Kindersley Limited
For further information see: www.dkimages.com

A WORLD OF IDEAS:
SEE ALL THERE IS TO KNOW

www.dk.com

CONTENTS

ACKNOWLEDGEMENTS

Thank you to everyone at DK Alpha Books for making this book possible. Special thanks to Brook, for meticulously editing each page and making sense of my drafts. To Becky, for her dazzling designs and perfect layouts. To Bill, for his organizational input and for keeping the project running. And to Mike, for his insight and for being a great publisher.

Thank you to my parents, Gail and Ira, for kicking me outside on a sunny day, instead of letting me watch TV. Thank you for involving me in athletics and teaching me to be a strong girl. You're a big reason why I grew into a strong woman.

Thank you to my boyfriend, Evan, for being my best friend and for being supportive.

Thank you to my favorites in the fitness industry—Brad Schoenfeld, Bret Contreras, Jacob Wilson, John Meadows, Rhonda Patrick, and Arnold Schwarzenegger. You have paved the way for the combination of science, healthy living, and smart training.

ABOUT THE AUTHOR

ERIN STERN is a professional bodybuilder and two-time Ms. Figure Olympia. She has won 14 IFBB (International Federation of Bodybuilding and Fitness) titles, including the 2012 Arnold Classic Europe, and has been featured on over 20 fitness and bodybuilding magazine covers. Erin has created training programs that have helped thousands of people reach their fitness and bodybuilding goals, with a mission to empower, educate, and enrich the lives of people through fitness and healthy living.

INTRODUCTION

YOU ARE A BODYBUILDER

Why did you pick up this book? Is your intent to radically change your physique? Is it to add some curves or muscle to your body? Whatever your answer may be, if you plan to use weights to reach your goal, then YOU are a bodybuilder. Bodybuilding gives you the ability to sculpt your body into your dream body, but whatever your goal may be—whether you plan to train for aesthetics with the goal of stepping onto a bodybuilding stage, or you just want to create impressive proportions and improve the way you look and feel—this book is for you.

LIFTING WEIGHTS CAN CHANGE YOU

The benefits of lifting weights go beyond just adding muscle. Focused training not only can change your physique, it can change your entire life. When you train your brain with strength training, it's rewired for the better; your balance will improve, you'll gain strength, and you'll sleep better. As you gain physical strength, you'll become stronger in all aspects of your life. If you're stressed, weights will be an impactful outlet. If you need a break from the outside world, weights will provide that respite. If you need to find a purpose, transforming yourself with weights will help illuminate your path.

I can personally attest to this. Growing up, I was a skinny, shy girl with low self-esteem. Running track at the collegiate level helped bolster my self-esteem, but I still didn't quite get "it" at that point. It took massive failures on personal, professional, and life levels for me to see the value in following a structured training plan and for it to make a significant impact on my life. When the rest of the world grew dim, I had the gym; it gave me an anchor, structure, purpose, and it enhanced my strength—both physically and mentally. I had no plans on competing when I started—I was simply working out as a way to escape my life temporarily—but lifting saved my life and gave me a new life.

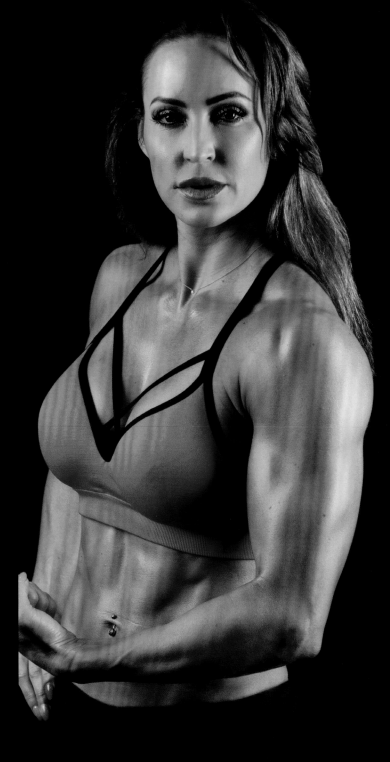

THIS BOOK WILL BE YOUR RESOURCE

The training programs, tips, and meal planning strategies in this book will enable success for people of all skill levels. You'll learn how to set objective goals, how to visualize those goals, and how to connect your mind and muscles to optimize each training day. You'll learn how to train properly and eat to gain muscle, maintain muscle, or lean down for definition. The meal plan strategies outline the important meals for the day and tell you how to eat for each one of the main training goals. Nine training plans ranging from four days per week to six days per week are designed to target specific muscle groups and will fit any schedule. You'll learn how to incorporate big compound lifts, nontraditional cardio, and nutrient timing into your training to make fast physique improvements, while spending less time in the gym doing it. The tips and techniques are sustainable, too, so you can continue to enjoy training and eating even after you complete a training program!

It's in us all to strive for improvement, but we often forget how important our health is. You've picked up this book, so now it's time to pick up some weights, and remember that every rep you perform will bring you closer to happiness, strength, and your ideal YOU!

Let's go train like a bodybuilder!

–Erin

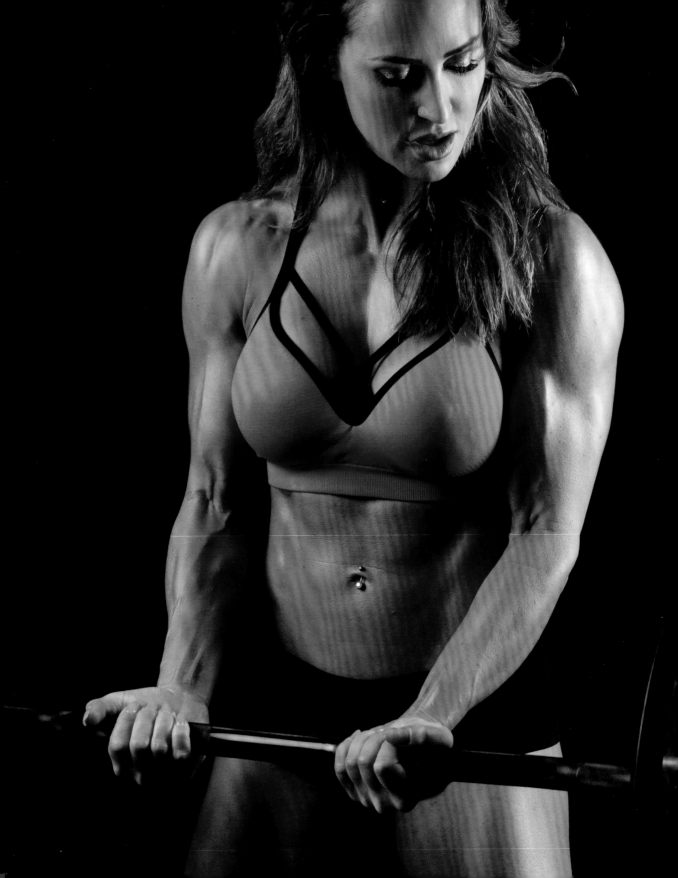

INTRODUCTION

WHY TRAIN LIKE A BODYBUILDER?

Training like a bodybuilder isn't about pushing tons of weight, it's about strategically sculpting your body to achieve a special look. It requires commitment, hard work, careful planning, and attention to detail.

THE BENEFITS

A sculpted bodybuilder body is unique, symmetrical, and a sight to behold, but strength training isn't all about gaining mass and pushing tons of weight. It's about training the body to be strong and balanced, and achieving a more complete level of fitness.

Fewer injuries Training for symmetry and aesthetics helps prevent injury by training all areas, and both sides of the body equally to eliminate weaknesses. Weight training also strengthens bones, so you're less prone to falling, and less apt to break something if you do fall. The result is a more complete level of strength.

A stronger, more balanced body Training for symmetry also helps improve body awareness and balance. As you train, your body will become more balanced from left to right, and from top to bottom. You'll increase both core strength and overall strength, so you'll no longer have a weak or strong side. Your body will be balanced and symmetrical, both in strength and in appearance.

A stronger brain and boosted metabolism It's no secret that strength training improves cognitive function, improves sleep, decreases stress, and improves immune health. The metabolic stress of lifting also increases your metabolism by increasing the mitochondria in your cells, which means your cells will be able to create more energy.

THE LOOK

What's special about the bodybuilder's body? It's about aesthetics and flow. The muscles tie together seamlessly and no muscle group looks out of place. It is art.

THE V-TAPER

The v-taper is that dramatic size differential between the upper back and the waist that you often see in bodybuilders. By training the right muscle groups, you can create the appearance of a smaller waist by strategically adding muscle to specific areas of the upper and lower body.

THE X-FRAME

An X-frame is defined by broad shoulders, a narrow waist, and muscular legs and glutes. Together they tie your upper body musculature together completely to make your waist appear smaller, and balance your physique from top to bottom. Lifters long for the X-frame and the superhero-like appearance it lends.

THE QUAD SWEEP

A strong, well-defined quad sweep not only adds thickness to the upper legs, but also adds curves to the outer portions of the upper legs. When quadriceps are well developed, they ripple with dimension and command attention with strong curves that are a sign of careful work in the gym.

THE CAPPED SHOULDERS

The shoulders are made up of three heads, and when all of the heads are trained properly, the result is capped shoulders that are perfectly rounded and tie in seamlessly to both the arms and the chest. They're the finishing touch on the ideal X-frame.

THE SIX-PACK

Attaining the perfect six-pack requires training every muscle in the abdominals while simultaneously cutting body fat to attain maximum definition. But when the abs are well developed, you'll be able to feel them and see them, and also notice a decrease in the circumference of your waist.

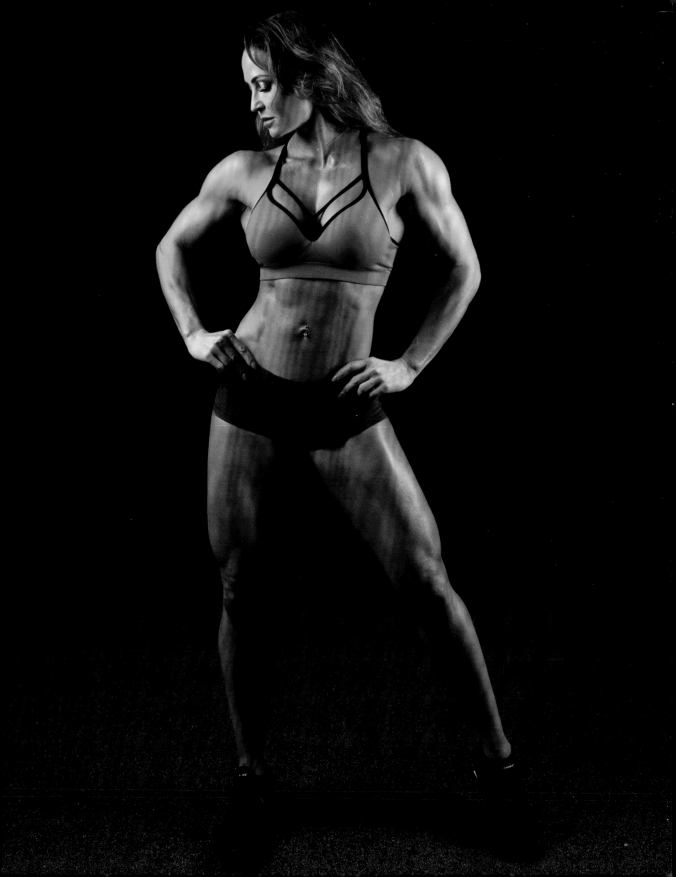

BASIC TYPES OF MOVEMENT

Bodybuilders train their muscles in a variety of ways. And by understanding the basic types of movement they employ to build muscle and train their bodies, and understanding how those movements benefit the body, you'll better understand how the workouts in this book work.

COMPOUND MOVEMENTS

Compound movements involve the engagement of multiple joints through the entire range of motion of an exercise. From an aesthetic viewpoint, compound movements help tie a physique together by training large muscle groups in unison. Most muscle-building training sessions should begin with compound movements, and more often than not you should opt for bigger compound movements over isolation movements to maximize the muscle-building effectiveness of your workouts. There are six basic lifts—squat, deadlift, bench, row, pull-up, and military press—and all are compound exercises, and each will be at the foundation of your workouts.

ISOLATION MOVEMENTS

Isolation exercises engage only one joint through the entire range of motion of an exercise. Biceps curls, triceps extensions, and leg extensions are all examples of isolation movements that will help sculpt or fine-tune only one muscle, or a small group of muscles. The "quad sweep," a smaller group of muscles located within the larger quadriceps, is an example of a small group of muscles that can be fine-tuned through isolation exercises.

NONTRADITIONAL CARDIO

Cardio is an important component of any muscle-building program, and nontraditional cardio techniques are the ideal way to add cardio to your training program—they're fun, challenging, and much harder for the body to adjust to than steady-state cardio activities. Nontraditional cardio creates a greater calorie burn than steady-state cardio, which means that less of your time will be spent in the gym on the cardio portion of your workouts. And because it's tougher for the body to adapt to training that changes frequently, there's less chance of hitting a training plateau. Following are some common nontraditional cardio methods you can integrate into your workouts.

HIIT

High-intensity interval training (HIIT) is the toughest form of nontraditional cardio, but it generates the best adaptations and quickest results. HIIT can involve a variety of exercises, but at its foundation it requires all-out effort for short bursts of exercise for 7 to 30 seconds, with only enough recovery time in between sets to allow your heart rate to drop to 60% of max. Your heart rate should reach 90% of max

ECCENTRIC AND CONCENTRIC MOVEMENTS

You may have heard the term "negatives" as it relates to weight training, and you will see this term used throughout this book. The negative, or *eccentric*, portion of an exercise is where the muscle lengthens during a movement. Conversely, when the muscle contracts during a movement, it does so during the *concentric* portion of the rep. A good example is a biceps curl: as you pull the weight toward you, the muscle is working concentrically, as you lower the weight back down to the starting position, the biceps is working eccentrically.

when measured immediately after a sprint, and sets should range from 4 to 8, depending on the complexity of the workout.

TABATA CIRCUITS

In addition to traditional HIIT, you'll find Tabata circuits in the workouts. A Tabata circuit is similar to a HIIT circuit, but is 4 minutes long and comprised of 8 rounds of all-out effort for 20 seconds, followed by 10 seconds of rest between rounds.

TIMED WORKOUTS

Timed workouts can be a challenging way to simply focus on each exercise. You can create a timed workout by choosing a time cap and then selecting the exercises to perform in a series or complex during that time cap, with some additional time built in for recovery. For example, you may choose to do 15 total minutes of 30 seconds each of burpees, lunges, jump rope, and jumping jacks, with 1 to 2 minutes of rest between each set. Timed workouts can be planned in any working ratio, but most use 1:1, 2:1, or 3:1 work-to-rest ratios.

FINISHERS

Just as the name implies, finishers are 5 to 10 minutes of high-intensity work that are done after your weight training session is complete. Finishers can help build mental toughness, burn fat, and help you see results more quickly. Medicine ball slams, shuttle runs, body weight circuits, and stair runs are all great examples of finishers. Finishers are best done after upper body training days, or on lighter leg days when your legs aren't completely fatigued from a vigorous training session. The work-to-rest ratio tends to be a bit higher for finishers: 3:1 or 4:1 works well, as the overall working time is lower compared to other forms of nontraditional cardio.

METABOLIC WORKOUTS

With metabolic workouts you choose a mix of high-intensity exercises and low-intensity exercises, and then combine them into timed circuits. The circuits can be anywhere from 30 seconds to 2 minutes, with recovery times in between sets ranging from 1 to 2 minutes. A sample metabolic workout might combine box jumps, burpees,

lunges, and planks. Or, you could combine sprint accelerations with lower-intensity moves like lunges. The total workout should take about 20 minutes, and can be performed after weight training or as a standalone workout.

STEADY-STATE CARDIO

Steady-state cardio activities, such as running, swimming, and biking are great tools for stress relief and active recovery, and also can help a bodybuilder lean down during the last 3 to 4 weeks of contest prep. However, because the body can quickly adapt to steady-state cardio, it's necessary to continuously increase the duration of the activity in order to continue to see benefits. It's for this reason that nontraditional cardio techniques are more effective and force the body to adapt more frequently. Nontraditional cardio also can improve metabolic flexibility, or the ability to burn both fats and carbs for fuel. If you do plan to integrate steady-state cardio into your program, you should perform it separately from your weight training sessions and opt for a stationary bike or stair climber, instead of the treadmill. Both of these machines focus more on concentric movement and hip flexion, so you won't get as sore, and you'll also be moving in ways that are more similar to how you'll be lifting.

HOW MUCH CARDIO **IS ENOUGH?**

When you're trying to build muscle, moderation is the key with all cardio. As a general rule, performing 1 to 2 days of nontraditional cardio during a training week is sufficient, and steady-state cardio should be limited to no more than 20 to 30 minutes per workout, and to no more than 1 to 2 days per week. Performing too much cardio can make it much harder to gain muscle, and it also can slow down recovery. Even if your goal is to only maintain muscle, performing too much cardio may actually lead to a decrease in muscle mass. If you're opting to include nontraditional or steady-state cardio in your plan, it's best to wait a few weeks before integrating it into your program so your body can adapt to the training.

STRENGTH TRAINING BASICS

There are a number of ways that muscle can be created when you strength train. By understanding these basic concepts and implementing the following techniques, you'll fine-tune your training and see results faster.

TEMPO

Tempo simply refers to the pace at which you move through a rep, and it can have a surprising impact on the effectiveness of strength training. Many lifters rush through sets without properly focusing on the muscle groups they're working. But when they're trying to gain or sculpt muscle, an experienced bodybuilder will slow down each rep and include a *one one thousand* count for each time they lower the weight, and an additional *one one thousand* count as they raise the weight back up. This helps increase tension on the muscle and also helps improve muscle awareness. Going more slowly with each rep also gives you time to feel the muscles working, and helps to maintain proper form.

FREQUENCY

Frequency simply refers to the number of times you can train per week (also known as a *split*). A few factors go into figuring out an optimal split, including your training goals, available time to train, level of fitness, and other factors. Ultimately, your goals and your lifestyle will determine how many times per week you'll need to train, but if you're looking to gain muscle, training five to six days per week is optimal. However, if you're just starting out, you may want to opt for training four days per week and then progressing to a higher frequency as you adapt. Whatever your goals may be, you should be realistic about how frequently you can train. If work or life is hectic and you can only manage to get to the gym four days per week, then you may need to adjust your goals. However frequently you do choose to train, it's best to hit every training session than to skip sessions due to an unrealistic split. Recovery can also be a factor in how frequently you can train. If you're still sore from a previous training session, you may be overtraining and may need to consider reducing your workout frequency until your body can adapt. Conversely, if you're not seeing the gains you want to see, you may not be training frequently enough and need to increase your frequency.

VOLUME

Training volume represents the number of reps you build into your workouts, and it can have a direct impact on muscle-building. Each muscle group requires the right amount of work to induce changes, and for muscle-building the "sweet spot" tends to be around 4 to 5 sets of 6 to 10 reps per exercise using heavy weight. For maintaining or leaning, the sets and reps will be slightly higher, but you'll be using less weight. Training volume should be high enough to cause adaptations, but not so extreme that your recovery is hindered. If you haven't recovered from a training session by the subsequent training session, you may be pushing too hard and may need to decrease the volume in your workouts.

TRAINING TECHNIQUES

There are a number of techniques that bodybuilders employ to improve their training and help maximize the effectiveness of their training.

Training to Failure (or AMRAP) Training to failure, or doing as many reps as possible (AMRAP), means you continue performing reps within a set until you simply can't do any more. This technique can help increase muscle fiber recruitment, create a greater ability to adapt to stress, and be valuable for developing toughness and improving progress, However, going to failure on compound exercises can cause damage that can take several days to recover from, so it's important to use this technique sparingly. (The programs in this book limit AMRAP to isolation movements and bodyweight exercises only.)

Isometric Holds Isometric holds are brief pauses at the shortest part of an exercise, or at maximum contraction. By pausing briefly at maximum contraction, you're able to bring more awareness to the area you're working and also increase the tension on the muscle, which can lead to better progress.

Partial Reps Muscles often can become accustomed to training through a full range of motion, which can result in training plateaus. Performing partial reps involves limiting the range of motion in a rep to either the top half of the rep, or the bottom half of the rep. Doing so can force muscles to adapt and help minimize plateaus that can result from muscles adapting to the full reps of an exercise.

Circuits A circuit, or metabolic workout, is another effective way to get the benefits of cardio while also using weights. In a circuit, four or more exercises are performed in succession, with the exercises being a combination of high-intensity and low-intensity exercises. The circuit is performed in a timeframe of 30 seconds to two minutes. Any combination of lifting and nontraditional cardio exercises will work.

Supersets By combining two exercises that work opposing muscle groups into one set (otherwise known as a *push-pull*), supersets can train antagonist, or opposing, muscle groups more efficiently than by doing standard sets. They can save time, improve strength, improve physique balance, prevent plateaus, and help you get the most out of a workout by allowing for more frequency throughout the week.

Compound Sets Compound sets can be used in two ways: by combining two exercises that train similar muscle groups, or by combining two exercises that use similar motions. Some examples might include combining lat pull-downs with rows (both working the back), or combining face pulls and biceps curls (both pulling motions).

Giant Sets Giant sets combine three exercises—often a mix of cardio and weight training—into one set, with the exercises performed in succession and without rest. These can save time, break plateaus, and also get the heart rate up since the exercises are performed back to back. Note that for promoting muscle growth, using isolation movements rather than compound movements is best for giant sets.

Pyramid Sets Pyramid sets decrease in the number of reps while increasing in weight as you progress through the set. Pyramid sets are modified to be lower in volume to allow you to train with high intensity for the full extent of the training session.

GRIP *STYLES*

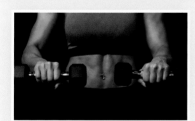

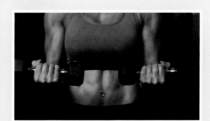

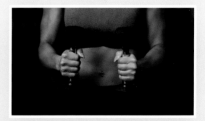

Overhand (pronated) Grasp the weight with your palms facing down. A *false* grip is an overhand grip without a thumb wrap. Some lifters prefer to use a false grip, but it can be dangerous, so you should always wrap your thumbs around the bar.

Underhand (supinated) Grasp the weight with your palms facing upward. Underhand grips are most commonly used for pulling exercises, and are particularly effective for training the biceps and the muscles in the front area of the shoulders.

Neutral Grasp the weights with your palms facing each other. This position can help take stress off of wrists, forearms, and shoulders. You can use a neutral grip when training with free weights or on machines, but not when using a bar.

HOW MUSCLE IS MADE

Your body's ability to repair and rebuild muscle tissue—and also create new muscle fibers—is a complex physiological process, but that process can be made more effective by paying attention to how you lift.

When muscles are stressed through strength training or other forms of strenuous exercise, the fibers in the muscles suffer microscopic tears. This damage is actually the beginning of the process that results in new muscle tissue being generated. When muscle fibers suffer these tears, the body's reaction is to repair or replace the torn fibers with new fibers that are thicker, which is why muscles grow in size when they're trained. These new fibers are called *myofibrils*, and the more you stress your muscles through weightlifting, the thicker and stronger these new fibers become. When the level of muscle generation (or muscle protein synthesis) is greater than the breakdown of muscle tissue, muscles grow larger. Contrary to popular belief, muscle protein synthesis doesn't actually happen during training—it happens during the rest and recovery stages. This is why adequate rest and recovery between training sessions is so essential to creating a well-designed strength-training program.

> **"**Contrary to popular belief, muscle protein synthesis doesn't actually happen during training—it happens during the rest and recovery stages. **"**

THE MECHANISMS OF BUILDING MUSCLE

How muscles grow is a complex physiological process that the body controls. But there are three key mechanisms that you can control as a lifter that can have a direct impact on the process of muscle protein synthesis.

ECCENTRIC EMPHASIS

As you train, you should pay close attention to always placing special emphasis on the negative, or *eccentric*, portion of every rep by performing the negative slowly. The negative is where the majority of the tears in muscle fibers occur during a movement, and since the muscle is considerably stronger in the negative portion of a rep compared to the concentric portion of the rep, performing the negative in a slow and controlled fashion will help encourage maximum change within the muscle. Research has shown that eccentric-focused training also helps recruit higher amounts of fast-twitch muscle fibers, which help lend a more athletic look to a physique.

MECHANICAL TENSION

Mechanical tension in the muscle occurs when you lift heavier weight, as opposed to lifting lighter weight. Compound movements are a great way to increase mechanical tension and maximize the benefits of your training. As a general rule, performing heavy sets in the 5 to 10 rep range for a muscle group is ideal for creating maximum muscle tension and promoting positive physique adaptations. Note that thresholds can vary from person to person, so use your best judgment when training. If your form starts to suffer and you can't perform the last 1 or 2 reps of a set, you should choose a lighter weight.

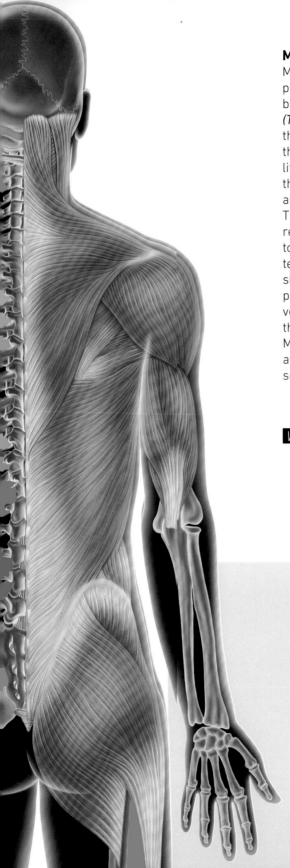

METABOLIC STRESS (OR *TUT*)

Metabolic stress essentially is the amount of time you place a muscle under stress during a rep. This concept became popular in the 1990s when it was coined *TUT (Time Under Tension)* by Charles Poliquin, and it means that the longer you can stress a muscle during a movement, the more benefit you're likely to gain from it. Quite often lifters will meticulously count the seconds as they control the weight through each rep, but for maximum TUT it's not as important to count as it is to perform each rep *slowly*. There are other ways you can increase TUT, including not relaxing the muscle at the top of a rep, or allowing gravity to take over at the bottom of a rep, both of which can take tension off the muscles. Increasing TUT also means you should increase the number of sets you perform as you progress through a workout, and choose a weight that is very challenging for the last few reps, but still light enough that you can keep proper form through the entire set. Maintaining proper form as the reps become difficult at the end of a set is critical, as this is where the muscle-sculpting really takes place.

WHY DO MUSCLES *GET SORE?*

Muscle soreness is caused by the micro-tears that occur in the muscle fibers during lifting, and DOMS (Delayed Onset Muscle Soreness) is the term used to describe this soreness. Lifters experience DOMS roughly 24 to 48 hours after a tough workout, and each lifter experiences the effects of DOMS differently, but it's not a negative result of strength training; it's actually a sign that your body is doing what it's supposed to be doing when you lift heavy weights—repairing existing muscle fibers and generating new muscle fibers. DOMS can be unsettling as you begin a training program, but the soreness will decrease as your body acclimates to the training. In the short term, you can treat DOMS with ice, stretching, massage, light activity, and plenty of rest. Pain relievers should be used only if absolutely necessary, as they can be detrimental to muscle growth and recovery.

DEVELOPING THE MIND-MUSCLE CONNECTION

Every successful bodybuilder has to master not only the physical side of bodybuilding, but the mental side, as well. By focusing your mind and utilizing the following techniques, you can make your training more efficient and effective, and also reach your training goals more quickly.

USING VISUALIZATION

Just as a sculptor wouldn't begin chiseling without a beautifully detailed end-result in mind, a bodybuilder never trains without being ever mindful of the end goal they've created in their mind's eye. Visualization is the mind-muscle connection that leads to materialization; which means that in order to create the physique you've always wanted, you first have to see it in your mind. You can start by simply closing your eyes and seeing your body, in detail, as you wish to see it. See the strong shoulders, broad chest, chiseled abs, and strong legs. Notice the details in your musculature and "feel" how strong you've become. Once you've created that clear vision of your goal in your mind, you're ready to integrate that visualization into your training. Before you begin your workouts, take a moment to revisualize the details of your ideal physique, and then continue to visualize your image between sets. Repeat your visualization even when you're not training to help keep your mind focused on the goal. This simple practice is the first step to developing the mind-muscle connection, and while it can take time and practice to master, it soon will become habit.

TRAINING WITH INTENTION

Training with intention involves using your senses to perfect your technique. One way to do this is by watching your *mirror muscles* as you train. Your mirror muscles are those you can see as you train, such as the biceps, shoulders, and quads. Watching your mirror muscles as you work them can help you improve your form and fine-tune your technique. A great exercise to practice this with is the leg extension. As you perform the leg extension, watch your quads closely and notice how they fire throughout the rep. As you slowly lower the weight back down, pay close attention to how your muscles are working. Are both legs firing evenly? Do you feel the outer or inner quads taking more of the load? Next, turn your toes in slightly and focus on lifting the weight with just your outer quads. Slowly raise the weight and watch the muscles working. Place your hands on your quads to feel the muscles working. Next, close your eyes and perform another slow rep, but this time using visualization to "see" the muscles working in your mind. Open your eyes and double check that your quads are firing the same way you were visualizing them firing. Turn your toes out just slightly and notice how your inner quad, or "teardrop," is firing. Keeping your toes straight on the next rep, try to isolate the teardrop in your mind and lift the weight with only the teardrop. Repeat this technique with other exercises and notice how slight changes in body angles and grips can target different parts of the muscles. By isolating and focusing on lifting the weight with just the intended area of each muscle, you can improve your results. The more awareness you bring into an exercise, the more aware you'll be as you train, and the more you'll improve your form. This technique may seem insignificant, but it can have a big impact

Training the muscles you *can't* see, such as the lats, glutes, and hamstrings, can be a little trickier, but it can be done by observing your muscles in a wall mirror and performing imaginary reps of an exercise. Observe how your muscles look and feel as you mimic the exercise. Watch your back as you squeeze your shoulder blades together. Mimic the motion of a lat pull-down by slowly pulling the imaginary weight to your chest. Vary the angles—leaning forward or leaning back—and make mental notes of how the muscles look and feel as you mimic the movements in the mirror. Now take these visualizations to the gym and replay them in your mind as you train the muscles you can't see. Concentrate on keeping your form tight and "seeing" them as you perform the rep. You'll soon notice the improvements in your form.

USING MINDFULNESS AND TRAINING "IN" THE MUSCLE

When you train, does your mind wander to other things? Or, do you keep your focus on the muscles you're working in the moment? By performing each rep with mindfulness and focusing on the intent to sculpt, you'll better master your form and see results more quickly. Every perfectly executed rep will bring you one step closer to your ideal physique, and by not allowing your mind to wander to other things as you perform each rep, you will better maintain your form and ensure that you're not recruiting other muscles to complete a set.

Training "in" the muscle is another important mind-muscle connection, and it simply means staying present during the last few tough reps of a set, which are the reps that happen to make the biggest difference in building a strong physique. Checking out or cheating during these final few critical reps can cause your form to suffer and induce fresher, stronger muscles to take over, which can limit the benefit. Always focus your efforts on moving the weight with just the intended muscles, and always finish your sets with intent and purpose.

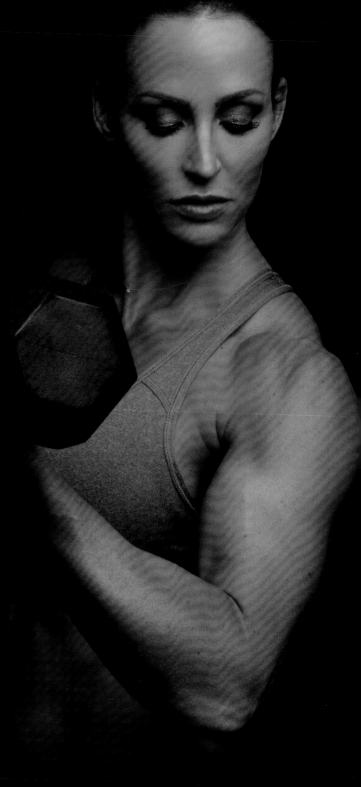

UNDERSTANDING MACROS

Everything you eat as a bodybuilder can be divided into two categories: macronutrients (or *macros*), which include protein, carbs, and fats; and micronutrients, which are the vitamins and minerals contained in the foods you consume. For bodybuilders, macros are what matter most.

PROTEIN

Protein is the building block of cells and should be eaten at every meal. When you consume protein, your body increases muscle protein synthesis to help build more muscle. And in order to increase muscle mass, or encourage the body to be in an anabolic state, consuming higher levels of dietary protein is critical. The typical diet averages about 0.36g of protein per pound of body weight, which equates to 54g of protein per day for a 150lb person, but a bodybuilder needs to consume much higher levels of protein to build muscle. The quality of the protein you consume also matters. Complete proteins, such as meats, fish, and eggs, contain all 21 essential amino acids, and also offer the best bioavailability, or ease of absorption. If you're on a vegan or vegetarian diet, you'll need to work a little harder to get enough protein to build muscle. Vegetarian protein sources, such as lentils and nuts, are less optimal because they offer lower bioavailability and don't contain complete amino acid profiles. Exceptions to this are hemp protein and protein powder blends that combine vegetarian sources while still providing more complete amino acid profiles.

CARBS

Carbohydrates serve two important purposes: they serve as fuel for your workouts, and they help repair and restore cells while you're at rest. Your body processes carbohydrates into glucose, which is what it then uses for fuel, and there are two types of carbs that each provide different forms of energy: simple and complex. Simple carbohydrates are digested quickly, are easy for the body to assimilate, and can aid in quick recovery after a tough workout, but the energy they provide is quickly depleted, so they're best consumed after a workout. Complex carbohydrates have higher levels of fiber and thus are digested more slowly, so they provide a more sustainable source of fuel for the body and are best consumed before a workout, when sustained energy is needed for the workout.

SOURCING YOUR NUTRIENTS

As a bodybuilder, carefully tracking your macro intake is one of the most important things you can do, but there are good sources of macros as well as some that should be avoided. Here are some examples of what to look for as you build your nutrition program and stock your kitchen.

PROTEIN

Complete protein sources: lean meats including chicken, beef, pork, fish, eggs, quinoa, Greek yogurt, and whey protein

Incomplete protein sources: peas, lentils, nuts and seeds, rice, legumes, whole wheat bread, peanut butter, and vegetables

FATS

For bodybuilders, consuming healthy dietary fats is important because they help repair cell damage that can occur through training, and they also help improve feelings of satiety. Brain health and mood are also boosted with adequate fat intake, and the immune system is bolstered, hair and skin health improve, and hormone production improves. Many important vitamins (like vitamins A, D, E, and K) need to be combined with fats for proper fat absorption, so it's important to get sufficient amounts of Omega 3, 6, and 9 fats in your diet to help with recovery. Note that dietary fat also is the easiest macro for the body to store as fat, so keep this in mind if you're actively bulking.

TEF *(THERMIC EFFECT OF FOOD)*

Metabolically, it takes considerable energy for the body to digest protein. This phenomenon is known as TEF, or the *Thermic Effect of Food*, and it can cause the body to burn up to five times more calories when it's digesting protein, compared to carbs or fats. With this in mind, you can increase your protein ratios and not only burn more calories, but also gain more muscle. It's also very difficult for the body to convert dietary protein into body fat, so if you're feeling hungry you can usually increase protein intake to increase feelings of satiety, and still maintain your diet.

HOW YOU COOK CAN MAKE A DIFFERENCE

- Cooking then cooling starches such as rice produces resistant starch, which means the starches can contain up to 30% fewer calories than fresh-cooked starches. Resistant starch is also more beneficial for gut health, so take this extra step when cooking starches.

- Most vegetable carbs, such as leafy greens, are "free" foods because they take more energy for the body to digest compared to the calories they provide.

- Most cooked vegetables contain a higher number of calories than when they're raw, since the cooking process releases more energy that the body can then use immediately. Your body has to work harder to digest raw vegetables.

- If you enjoy red meat well done, you'll be consuming more calories than someone who eats red meat that's been cooked rare or medium rare. Cooking denatures protein and, in a way, does some of the digesting for you, so your body doesn't have to work as hard to digest it. Cooking red meat less means your body will have to work harder to digest it, and that's a good thing.

CARBS

Complex (good) carb sources: whole grains, brown rice, legumes, sweet potatoes, low-sugar fruits (citrus, berries, and kiwifruit)

Simple carb sources: high-sugar fruits (grapes, bananas, and watermelon), baked goods and cereals, refined or raw sugar, and fruit juices

FATS

Sources of healthy fats: tree nuts, nut butters, olive oil, eggs, chia seed, flax seed, full-fat dairy, oily fish (salmon, tuna), and avocados

Fat sources to avoid: processed meats, margarine, and highly processed oils (corn, soybean, sunflower, vegetable, cottonseed)

CHOOSING A NUTRITION PLAN

Nutrition plays a significant role in the success of every training program. Once you've decided on your training goals, it's time to choose a nutrition plan that will align with those goals and help you identify your daily macro needs.

BULKING PLAN (30/40/30)

A bulking plan is the fastest way to gain muscle. With that said, eating for bulking doesn't mean you can eat everything in sight; you'll still need to carefully manage your macros to ensure you're getting the right balance to maximize muscle growth. Also, note that you can gain fat while on a bulking plan, so a bulking phase may need to be followed by a leaning phase in order to lose some of the fat added during the bulk. If you're struggling to gain muscle during a bulking phase, add additional calories to your daily macros in 5% increments until you begin to see results.

DAILY MACROS AND CALORIES

Fat (30%): A higher ratio of fat is needed for recovery and rebuilding.

Carbs (40%): A high ratio of carbs is essential since the body needs carbs for fuel and recovery, and to help with building muscle.

Protein (30%): To gain muscle, you should consume 1.5g–2g of protein per pound of body weight, per day.

Calories (+15% variance): You should plan to always be in a 15% caloric surplus over your daily maintenance calories to encourage muscle protein synthesis and avoid muscle breakdown throughout the day.

CLEAN BULKING PLAN (20/40/40)

A clean bulking plan can take longer to have an effect than a traditional bulk, but it often doesn't require a leaning phase at the end to trim any fat gained during the bulk. While following a clean bulking plan, pay close attention to nutrient timing to ensure you're getting sufficient protein and carbs both before and after training sessions. Also, be sure to carefully manage your portion sizes since your caloric intake will need to be lower than it would be with a traditional bulk.

DAILY MACROS AND CALORIES

Fat (20%): A lower dietary fat intake than a standard bulk provides an additional leaning component.

Carbs (40%): A high ratio of carbs is essential since the body needs carbs for fuel, recovery, and building muscle.

Protein (40%): You should consume 1–1.5g of protein per pound of body weight, per day. If the results aren't satisfactory, adjust your protein intake upward every 7 to 10 days until you start seeing the results you're seeking.

Calories (+10% variance): You should stay closer to maintenance levels, but run a slight caloric surplus particularly before and after training to encourage muscle growth.

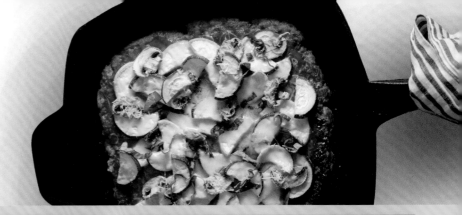

MAINTENANCE PLAN (30/30/40)

To maintain muscle, you should monitor overall ratios and food intake on a weekly basis and adjust intake based on your activity levels to ensure you keep hard-earned muscle. Making weekly adjustments and increasing, or decreasing, caloric intake to match your daily activity levels (known as *calorie cycling*) will help you avoid plateaus, and can also help you avoid a dieter's mindset of scarcity.

DAILY MACROS AND CALORIES

Fat (30%): A higher fat intake will help you recover from tough workouts, and also help you fend off hunger.

Carbs (30%): You'll still need a high ratio of carbs for training and recovery—just not as much as you would for a bulk or clean bulk.

Protein (40%): Protein intake should remain higher than normal, so you should consume about 0.8g–1g of protein per day, per pound of body weight. You will need to keep protein intake high to prevent muscle breakdown during training.

Calories (-5% variance on rest or light days/ 0% variance on heavy training days): Run a slight caloric deficit on rest or light training days, then follow maintenance calories on heavy training days.

LEANING PLAN (20/30/50)

A leaning plan also uses calorie cycling to help prevent the muscle loss and plateau that often can accompany low-calorie diets. You'll adjust your caloric intake depending on when and how hard you train. If you find you're struggling to lose fat while on a leaning plan, try adding additional cardio to your workouts, but don't be tempted to cut additional calories beyond the recommended variances. Cutting too many calories can send your body into starvation mode, which can stall your progress.

DAILY MACROS AND CALORIES

Fat (20%): A low dietary fat intake provides an important leaning component.

Carbs (30%): While carb intake is slightly lower, it's still high enough to fuel your workouts and help you recover.

Protein (50%): You should keep your protein intake high at 1–1.5g of protein per pound of body weight, per day, The high protein intake can improve satiety, and help prevent your body from entering a catabolic state.

Calories (-10% variance on rest or light days/ 0% variance on heavy training days): Run a higher caloric deficit on rest or light training days, then follow maintenance calories on heavy training days.

CALCULATING YOUR DAILY MACROS

Once you've selected a nutrition plan, you need to calculate your daily macro needs. And while a lot of bodybuilders often obsess over calories, tracking macros is more flexible, easier to manage, and more effective than counting calories.

STEP 1: DETERMINE YOUR DAILY MAINTENANCE CALORIES

Maintenance calories are what your body needs each day to maintain current weight, based on sex, current weight, current activity level, and other factors.

*(**Note:** These tables provide only general calorie recommendations. For more accurate calorie targets that are specific to your personal needs and specifications, it's recommended you access an online calculator to generate your specific calorie targets.)*

Low active: You train 1–2 days per week, and your workouts are low- to moderate-intensity.

Moderate active: You train 2–3 days per week, and your workouts are low- to moderate-intensity.

High Active: You train 4–5 days per week, and your workouts are moderate- to high-intensity.

Very high active: You train 5–6 days per week, and your workouts are high-intensity.

WOMEN
(ESTIMATED CALORIES FOR A 5'4" 32-YEAR-OLD FEMALE)

WEIGHT	LOW ACTIVE	MODERATE ACTIVE	HIGH ACTIVE	VERY HIGH ACTIVE
80	1166	1377	1589	1800
90	1216	1436	1657	1877
100	1265	1495	1725	1955
110	1315	1554	1793	2032
120	1365	1613	1861	2109
130	1415	1672	1929	2186
140	1465	1731	1997	2263
150	1515	1790	2065	2340
160	1565	1849	2133	2417
170	1615	1908	2201	2494
180	1665	1967	2269	2571
190	1715	2026	2337	2649

MEN
(ESTIMATED CALORIES FOR A 5'10" 32-YEAR-OLD MALE)

WEIGHT	LOW ACTIVE	MODERATE ACTIVE	HIGH ACTIVE	VERY HIGH ACTIVE
110	1603	1894	2185	2476
120	1653	1953	2253	2553
130	1703	2012	2321	2630
140	1752	2071	2389	2707
150	1802	2130	2457	2784
160	1852	2189	2525	2861
170	1902	2248	2593	2939
180	1952	2307	2661	3017
190	2002	2365	2729	3093
200	2052	2424	2797	3170
210	2102	2483	2865	3247
220	2152	2542	2933	3324

NOT ALL CALORIES *ARE* CREATED EQUALLY

Every calorie is a unit of energy, but not all calories are created equally, and different types of foods have different caloric measures. While protein and carbs each contain 4 calories per gram, fats are more nutrient-dense at 9 calories per gram. Once you've calculated your total daily calories for each macro, you can use those numbers to calculate your total daily gram allowances for each macro.

STEP 2: CALCULATE YOUR DAILY MACRO NEEDS

Once you've determined your daily calories needs, you need to calculate your daily macro needs based on the nutrition plan you've chosen. You can do so by doing some simple math. Here's an example:

Sample: High active 140lb female following a bulking nutrition plan

The total daily calories needed to maintain her current weight is 2263. For a bulking program, the daily caloric variance is an additional 15%, so her total daily calorie allowance is now **2602** (2263 x 1.15).

The macro ratio for a bulking program is 30/40/30 (30% fats/40% carbs/30% protein), so she can take her total calories and multiply them by these percentages to calculate her total calorie allowances for each macro:

Fat: (2602 x .3) = 781 calories
Carbs: (2602 x .4) = 1041 calories
Protein: (2602 x .3) = 781 calories

Now that she's calculated her calorie percentages, she can calculate the total daily grams of each macro based on the caloric values of each macro (1 gram of fat = 9 calories, 1 gram of carbs = 4 calories, 1 gram of protein = 4 calories):

Fat: 781 calories / 9 = 87 grams
Carbs: 1041 calories / 4 = 260 grams
Protein: 781 calories / 4 = 195 grams

The overall daily macro needs for a high active 140lb female following a bulking program are:

87 grams of fat per day
260 grams of carbs per day
195 grams of protein per day

Once you know your daily macros, you'll no longer need to count every calorie; you can simply track the total grams of each macro you consume each day.

TIPS FOR MEAL PLANNING SUCCESS

- **Be flexible** Remember that meal planning and tracking ratios is part science, part art, and part guesswork, so be flexible in your approach until you find the ratios that work best for you

- **Make sensible, healthy food choices** Try to eat meals that consist mostly of single-ingredient foods.

- **Keep meals simple and watch your portions** You won't have to worry about small fluctuations in calories

- **Eat the right meal combinations** Eat meals that are primarily combinations of proteins and fats or proteins and carbs, and avoid eating meals that feature an overabundance of fats and carbs

- **Consume the bulk of your carbs and calories around training sessions** You'll maximize the benefits of your nutrient intake and better fuel your workouts

- **Increase healthy fat intake when decreasing carb intake** Your body will better utilize the fats to aid in the healing of existing muscle and also aid in the generation of new muscle tissue

- **Keep a food journal** Tracking meals and daily macro intake will improve your results. And don't stress if you're off target by a few grams—the body is amazingly adaptive and can adjust, whether you're slightly under or slightly over

- **Reassess your progress every 7 to 10 days** Your macro ratios may change as your body changes, so don't be afraid to make adjustments if you begin to stall on your current plan

EATING FOR MUSCLE GAIN

Maximizing your muscle gains in the gym begins with understanding how your body processes the fuel you put in it, and optimizing when and how you eat to help you better fuel your workouts.

UNDERSTANDING ANABOLIC AND CATABOLIC STATES

At any given time, your body is in one of two metabolic states: anabolic or catabolic. When it's in an anabolic state, it's actively repairing muscle tissue damaged during workouts and creating new muscle tissue. When it's in a catabolic state, however, the body is actively breaking down muscle tissue. So, in order to grow or even maintain hard-earned muscle tissue, your body needs to be in an anabolic state more often than it's in a catabolic state, and your body needs energy for anabolism to take place. By feeding your muscles the right nutrients at the right times, you'll optimize the benefits gained during training and also aid recovery and rebuilding. Lifting heavy weights, utilizing compound movements, and keeping most of your reps in a range of 6 to 12 per set also will help keep your body in an anabolic state. You can avoid entering a catabolic state by avoiding excessive cardio, particularly steady-state cardio, during your training week, and limiting your weight workouts to one hour or less.

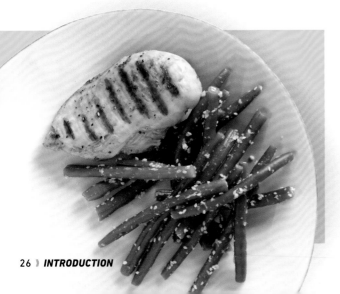

MEAL FREQUENCY AND TIMING

Meal frequency simply refers to how many times per day you eat. The traditional belief among lifters was that you needed to eat multiple small meals throughout the day, and in 2 to 3 hour intervals, to keep the body in an anabolic state. However, more recent studies have shown that eating 3 to 4 larger meals per day is just as effective, as long as each meal contains the right ratios of protein, carbs, and healthy fats to promote muscle building.

Additionally, *when* you eat your meals is just as important for maximizing the nutrients you consume. Meals should be timed to be eaten mostly before and after workouts, when nutrients can be best used for fuel and recovery. You should avoid eating meals late in the day when your body is at rest and preparing for sleep. Our bodies follow a circadian rhythm, which is a 24-hour cycle that's influenced by light, darkness, and our own internal clocks. This natural clock also controls your brain waves, hormone production, and cell regeneration, and as it nears time to sleep, your metabolism slows, your blood pressure decreases, and your body releases melatonin to signal sleep. Your metabolism is interconnected with your circadian rhythms, and since your metabolism is highest during the day and when you're active, most of your calories should be consumed at these times. Eating before going to bed means excess calories can more easily be stored as fat, and sleep and recovery can be disrupted. As you awaken, your body releases adrenaline and cortisol to prepare for activity, increasing your metabolism. Consuming most of your calories earlier in the day and around the times you're most active means you'll be maximizing the fuel you feed your body, and you'll also sleep better, train harder, and get leaner.

PRE-WORKOUT NUTRITION

What you eat before you train will be the fuel you use to power through your workout. About 1.5 to 2 hours before training, you should eat a meal comprised primarily of lean protein and complex carbs. The protein will encourage muscle protein synthesis and the complex carbs will help bolster energy stores and provide sustained energy to fuel your workout. By following this simple approach you'll find you have good energy to maintain lifting intensity and focus. You should avoid consuming overly acidic foods like citrus, as well as fatty foods, spicy foods, and dairy before training sessions, as these foods are harder to digest and may cause stomach problems during training. As a general rule, lean proteins should be included with every snack, and you should increase your carb consumption both before and after training, while keeping healthy fat intake relatively low.

POST-WORKOUT NUTRITION

After a hard workout you will have burned through most of your energy stores, so you should consume faster-digesting proteins and simple carbs to help speed recovery and promote the building and rebuilding of muscle fibers. The carbs will help decrease cortisol, a stress hormone that is released during strenuous exercise. Cortisol can be catabolic, so consuming carbs after training can help prevent any muscle loss that may occur due to an increased level of cortisol in your body. Post-workout meals should include faster-digesting carbs and easy-to-assimilate sources of protein like fresh fruit, rice cakes, protein shakes, Greek yogurt, chicken breasts, or low-fat milk to help replenish energy stores and aid in muscle building and recovery. A good, simple post-workout meal might include a whey protein shake and a serving of fruit, or a serving of light Greek yogurt and fruit.

When you're in a more sedentary state, you should decrease carb consumption and increase healthy fat intake to aid in the recovery and repair of muscle tissue. Fats can help with satiety and have no impact on insulin, so they're ideal to consume when the body is more sedentary. When you're sedentary, carb intake should be very minimal or eliminated. Simply put: as the intensity of your workouts increases or decreases, your calorie and carb intake should be adjusted accordingly. Think of carbs as fuel in a car—you wouldn't overfill the tank just to let the car sit in the driveway, so you shouldn't overfeed your body if you don't plan on training with intensity.

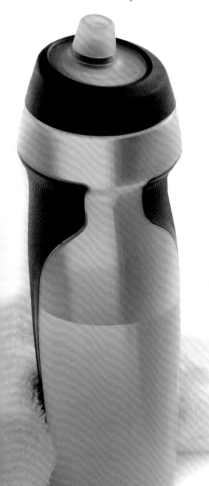

> **❝** Think of carbs as fuel in a car— you wouldn't overfill the tank just to let the car sit in the driveway, so you shouldn't overfeed your body if you don't plan on training with intensity. **❞**

NUTRITION SUPPLEMENTS

Supplements should always be considered just that: supplements to a healthy, balanced diet. But if you're looking for additional tools that can aid in recovery, muscle-building, and overall healthy functioning, supplements can help.

PROTEIN SHAKES

Protein shakes can be beneficial when used as a post-workout nutrition boost, as a meal replacement during bulking, or in a pinch when you don't have time for a meal. When shopping for protein shakes, choose faster-digesting protein post-workout options like a hydrolyzed isolate or a whey isolate. These options are lactose-free and can be good options for those who are adversely affected by lactose. If you are bulking, a whey blend might be more beneficial and will have several forms of protein ranging from fast- to slow-digesting. (In order of speed of digestion, isolate is the fastest, followed by concentrate and casein [Note that both concentrate and casein can contain lactose.]).

When choosing a protein powder, look for one that has a protein serving that's very close to the overall serving weight. For example, if a scoop serving is 30g, but contains only 22g of protein, that could mean that there are unnecessary fillers included in the powder. Note that some protein powders may also contain carbs or fat, in which case you should subtract the carbs and fat grams from the serving total to determine if there are any unnecessary fillers. The goal is to find a protein powder that has a protein serving that is close to the scoop serving size. This will limit the amount of fillers you consume that won't contribute to nutrition or gains.

CAFFEINE

Caffeine can be beneficial as a pre-workout supplement. Take around 200mg, 30 minutes before training, to boost exercise performance and give you energy. Black coffee or caffeine tablets both work well. Be sure to start with a low dose to first assess your sensitivity.

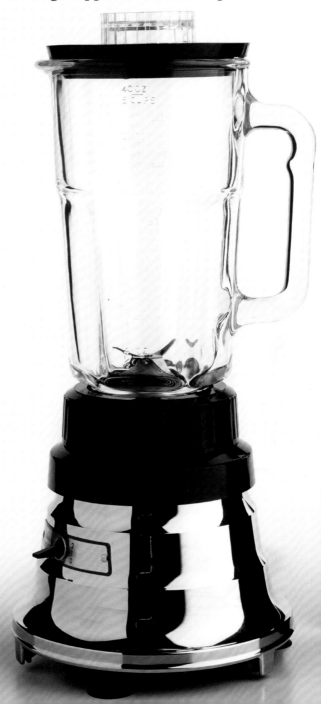

CREATINE MONOHYDRATE

Still referred to as the "gold standard" for gaining muscle, creatine is beneficial for both increasing muscle mass and improving strength. There are many forms of creatine, but creatine monohydrate remains the most studied, least expensive, and most effective. It's a budget-friendly choice, as well. There is no need to load creatine, you can simply add 2–5g to a daily post-workout shake. The sugars in the powder will help your body absorb it.

CHELATED MAGNESIUM OR MAGNESIUM GLYCINATE

Magnesium is present in every cell of the body, and the body needs it to maintain all functions. However, intense training, lack of sleep, or stress can deplete the body of magnesium, so you might want to consider taking a magnesium supplement. The benefits of taking a magnesium supplement may include better sleep, better recovery, improved digestion, boosted exercise performance, and improved muscle gain. Chelated or buffered magnesium, or magnesium glycinate, can all help replenish magnesium levels without causing stomach upset.

VITAMIN D3

Also known as the "sunshine vitamin," vitamin D3 bolsters immunity, can aid in weight loss, can improve bone health, and can help improve athletic performance. Many people are deficient in this vitamin, and the FDA recommended amount is rather low. So if you're not out in the sun often, a daily dose of up to 10,000 IU can result in drastic improvements in your health and training.

OMEGA 3

Supplementing with Omega 3 can help reduce inflammation, improve insulin sensitivity, reduce free radicals, enhance skin and hair health, and improve joint health. The most popular supplement is a fish oil containing both EPA and DHA, two polyunsaturated fatty acids. Choose a dose that is around 2,000 mg for both, and look for brands that are purity-tested and mercury-free.

CURCUMIN

Curcumin, an extract of turmeric, can greatly reduce inflammation and improve immune system function.

PRODUCTS TO AVOID

- The supplement industry isn't heavily regulated, so you should avoid supplements that aren't certified. Look for supplements from third party-verified companies that include "certified safe for sport" or "informed choice" logos on their products, to ensure quality and purity.

- Avoid generic multivitamins, as the vitamins and minerals tend to be mostly man-made, and the body doesn't recognize them, which often means the ingredients can simply pass through the body, rather than being absorbed.

- Avoid supplements that claim to boost hormones. These can have the opposite effect and can throw the body out of balance.

- Steer clear of fat burners, especially those containing ingredients like *yohimbe* or *rauwolscine (alpha-yohimbine)*. Negative side effects of fat burners can include dizziness, rapid heartbeat, nausea, and trouble sleeping.

- Avoid products that contain artificial colors like FD&C red or blue, and avoid fillers like titanium dioxide (a whitening agent) or potassium sorbate (a preservative), as these can potentially cause harm or irritation.

Look for a supplement that contains bioperine or black pepper extract, as these ingredients can help with absorption. If you can't find curcumin, use can use organic turmeric and black pepper in your cooking to get some of the same benefits.

GLUTAMINE

Glutamine is a semi-essential amino acid the body needs to function, and it can be beneficial for recovery after training and also for maintaining gut health. Although your body makes glutamine, it can quickly be leached out of the your system through intense training or stress. 5g a day in a post-workout shake can aid in recovery from particularly tough training sessions.

AROUND THE GYM (EQUIPMENT)

Every gym is a bit unique, but most gyms still contain the same basics tools for training. By familiarizing yourself with some of the most common equipment used in weight training gyms, you'll be able to train harder and smarter.

BARS

Olympic bar This standard 45lb straight bar can be used with or without weights. If you're performing heavy exercises, the bar can be secured at the squat rack or placed on the gym floor. You can also place one end in a sturdy corner to perform endless back, legs, and accessory exercises.

EZ bar The EZ bar is a curved bar that may be empty, or may be pre-loaded with weights. The standard empty EZ bar ranges from 15 to 25lb, while pre-loaded EZ bars can range from 20lb to up over 100lb. Pre-loaded bars will be labeled on the sides of the plates for easy identification.

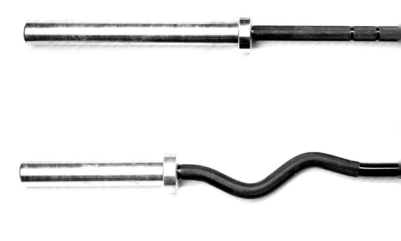

MACHINES

Cable machine The cable machine is the most versatile training tool in the gym and is used for everything from lat pull-downs to cable rows. The standard cable machine includes brackets or pins for adjusting the cables to varying heights in order to target different areas of the body. Different attachments help expand the usefulness of this essential machine.

Smith machine The Smith machine is a great tool for guided range of motion and self-spotting exercises. The bar, usually weighing 15lb is attached to the machine on a fixed plane of motion and can be directly perpendicular to the floor or angled slightly. Pegs on each side allow you to adjust the range of motion upward or downward.

Leg extension machine This machine is recognizable by an elevated seat along with a left- or right-hand padded lever that runs parallel to, and directly below, the seat. You can adjust the lever up or down, depending on your height. If there's a seat, you can adjust it backward or forward to fit your range of motion. Adjust the weight by placing a pin below the plate of your choice.

Leg curl machine This machine comes in two varieties: lying or seated. The lying leg curl machine is the most common and is recognizable by its slightly v-shaped pad with a padded lever at one end and handles at the other. The lever adjusts closer or farther from the pad to allow for height differences. It also adjusts up or down to control range of motion.

CABLE MACHINE ATTACHMENTS

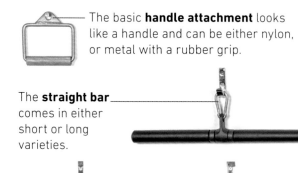

The basic **handle attachment** looks like a handle and can be either nylon, or metal with a rubber grip.

The **straight bar** comes in either short or long varieties.

The **EZ bar attachment** is curved like the free-weight EZ bar.

The **v-bar** is a metal bar that's shaped like a "V".

The **double-D handle** has two metal handles that come together in a "V" shape.

The **rope attachment** is a long nylon rope that's secured to the cable in the middle.

OTHER EQUIPMENT

Adjustable bench The adjustable bench can accommodate every exercise requiring the use of a bench. The bench will have knobs for adjustments, and some benches will automatically raise the incline of the seat, while others will have a pin below the seat to adjust the seat height or incline.

Squat rack This gym staple allows you to lift heavy weights more safely. The rack has incremental "J" hooks for placing the Olympic bar at a suitable height for racking and re-racking. Adjustable cross pins allow you to set maximum bar depth for various exercises, and also add an additional layer of safety. Some gyms have what is called a "power rack," which does not include the cross pins.

Dip chair This machine looks like a giant chair without a seat and is sometimes called a Roman chair. There are padded arms on either side of the seat, and rubberized pegs with grips at the end of each arm. Raised foot platforms on either side help you get into a good position for performing ab work or dips.

Calf raise machine This machine comes in two varieties: seated or standing. The seated version features a seat with a foot platform below and knee pads above, with an upright rack to hold plates and a safety lever which must be pushed to the side when you're secured in the machine. The standing version has an elevated foot platform with adjustable shoulder rests and an adjustable weight.

Leg Press The leg press has a large seat and a large foot platform. Plates can be loaded on either side of the machine, and calf raises often can be performed without removing the safety levers, but always pay careful attention to the unloaded sled, which can weigh from 45 to 110lb.

WEIGHTS

Plates Plates come in standard 2.5lb, 5lb, 10lb, 25lb, and 45lb sizes, and are made to fit on the Olympic bar. Additionally, plates can be used in lieu of dumbbells, as anchors for exercises like t-bar rows, or stacked to make small steps to increase range of motion. Plates are typically made from steel, while others may be made from rubber (typically referred to as *bumper plates*).

Dumbbells Dumbbells are the most-utilized tools in the gym. They come in pairs and can range from 2lb to over 100lb each. Most gyms will have designated racks for the dumbbells, where they will be sorted in ascending order.

KNOW YOUR MUSCLES

Understanding the basic musculature in your body is an essential part of being a bodybuilder.

This guide will help you learn where the major muscle groups in the body are located, as well as where smaller muscles are located within the larger muscle groups.

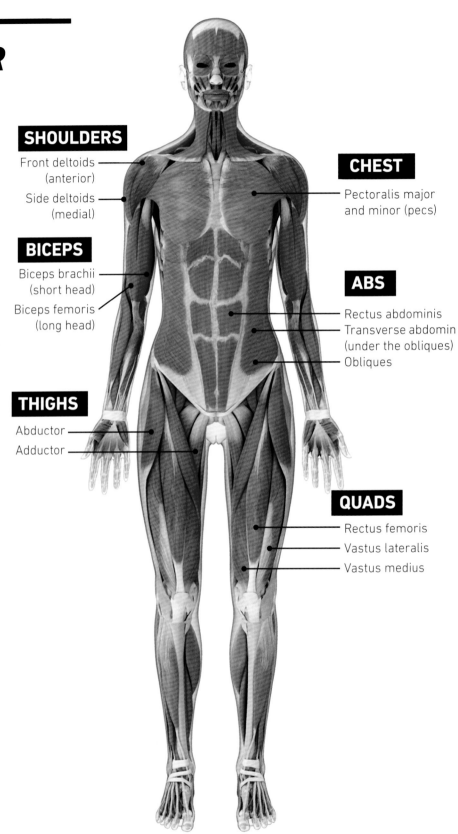

SHOULDERS
Front deltoids (anterior)
Side deltoids (medial)

BICEPS
Biceps brachii (short head)
Biceps femoris (long head)

THIGHS
Abductor
Adductor

CHEST
Pectoralis major and minor (pecs)

ABS
Rectus abdominis
Transverse abdomin (under the obliques)
Obliques

QUADS
Rectus femoris
Vastus lateralis
Vastus medius

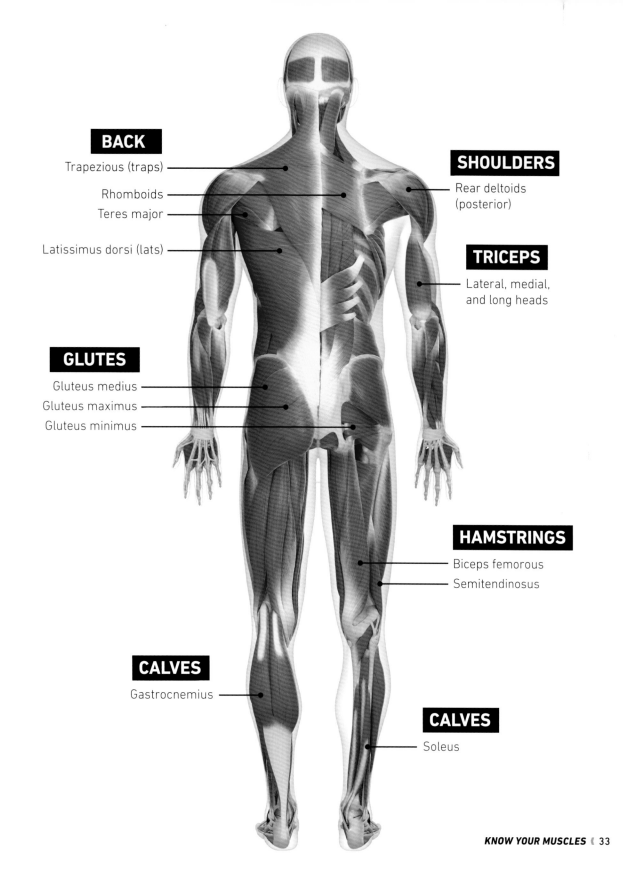

BACK

Trapezious (traps) ——

Rhomboids ——

Teres major ——

Latissimus dorsi (lats) ——

SHOULDERS

Rear deltoids (posterior)

TRICEPS

Lateral, medial, and long heads

GLUTES

Gluteus medius ——

Gluteus maximus ——

Gluteus minimus ——

HAMSTRINGS

Biceps femorous

Semitendinosus

CALVES

Gastrocnemius ——

CALVES

Soleus

TIPS FOR SMARTER TRAINING

Proper strength training has less to do with the amount of weight you lift, and more to do with *how* you lift. Observing these best practices will help you build muscle and reach your training goals faster. Perfect practice makes perfect, and over time these actions will become habits.

STRIVE FOR SYMMETRY

As you train, make sure that both sides of the body are pushing or pulling evenly, and that your weight is distributed evenly. Start with your weaker side and then move on to the stronger side, and perform the same number of reps that you did on your weaker side.

WATCH YOUR FORM

Paying close attention to your body during each exercise can result in better progress and fewer injuries. For example, keeping your core tight will not only help you build beautiful abs, but it will also help protect your back. Keeping your spine neutral will help take pressure off of your back, and ensure years of injury-free training. Keeping your feet flat and even, and keeping your wrists straight when pulling or pushing weight, will ensure your body is always in balance as you train.

VARY YOUR GRIPS

A slight change in grips can change an entire exercise. For example, switching your grip from an overhand to an underhand grip on a row can mean you go from targeting your back to targeting your biceps. By incorporating a variety of grips into your training, you'll hit muscles from all angles and better improve your strength and overall aesthetics. You also can adjust your grip widths to further increase the variety in your lifts, which also will help you avoid plateaus while still keeping workouts challenging.

EMPLOY CONTROLLED CHEATING AND SELF-SPOTTING

Controlled cheat reps are a great way to train muscles through their strongest range of motion: the negative. With this strategy, you use momentum, gravity, or power from otherwise non-contributing muscles to help you power through the concentric portion of the rep, while still controlling the more important negative portion of the rep. This allows you to get a few more forced reps in at the end of a set, which can ultimately lead to more size and strength gains. Choose your cheat reps wisely, though; this strategy works best on isolation movements like pull-ups, the standing shoulder press, or seated rows, but should not be used during movements like the squat, deadlift, or bench press.

Self-spotting can be used to boost the last few reps in a set by assisting a rep with a non-working arm. For the upper body, you can use a free hand to help with the last few reps by spotting the concentric (negative) portion of the rep. For the lower body, you can self-spot a leg press by pushing your hands against your upper leg. Pulling up on the handles of the seated calf raise also will help you squeeze in a few more negatives. Self-spotting works well for certain isolation movements, like single-arm biceps curls, the leg press, seated calf raise, or single-arm triceps extensions.

Note that these strategies are useful, but shouldn't be relied upon for every workout. Aim to add them in once or twice a week, or when you might be struggling to complete sets.

DON'T OVERSTIMULATE YOUR CENTRAL NERVOUS SYSTEM (CNS)

The body can't handle high volumes of training day after day, and the central nervous system takes about twice as long to recover as the muscles do. For natural athletes, recovery is a bit slower than it is for enhanced athletes, so techniques like training to failure should be limited to finishers, or used only on isolation exercises to limit central nervous system (CNS) fatigue. To further avoid CNS fatigue, pay careful attention to how you feel before, during, and after you train, particularly after you've completed two to three tough training sessions in a row. If you feel foggy, have trouble sleeping, experience nagging aches and pains, or if the weights feel heavier than they should, consider going easy for a few days. Plan a deload week every four to six weeks to help your body recover fully and to help keep you in top lifting form. A deload week is a week of lighter activity to allow the body to recover from heavy training. Nagging aches and pains and overall fatigue can be eliminated with a deload, which might include circuit training in the gym supplemented with light weights, stretching, and active recovery through activities like walking and swimming. Remember that rest repairs muscle, while the gym tears muscle down. Listen to your body and work toward stimulating the muscles to grow. (It's a good mental break, too.)

STAY SAFE IN THE GYM

When you're in the gym, always use clips and collars when securing plates onto bars, and never perform any exercises without a clip positioned snugly at each end of the bar and against the plates. Additionally, when loading plates onto an Olympic or EZ bar, never overload one side of the bar, and always match the weight from one side to the other as you load the plates. Finally, and importantly, never perform any exercises that require a spotter, if you don't have a spotter to assist.

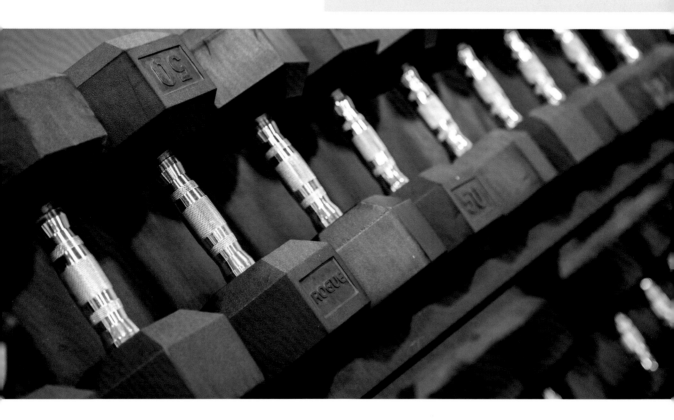

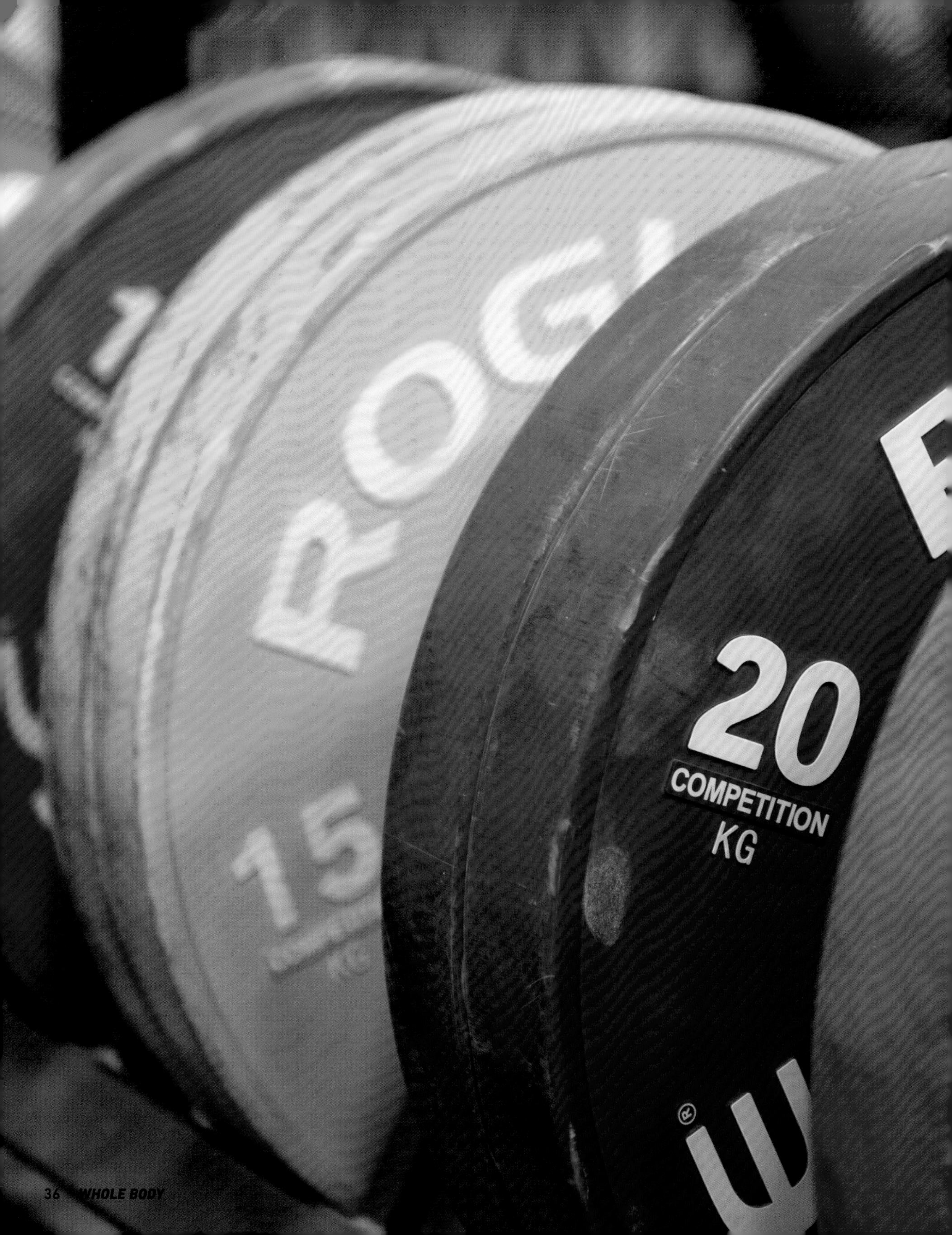
ROG
15
20
COMPETITION
KG

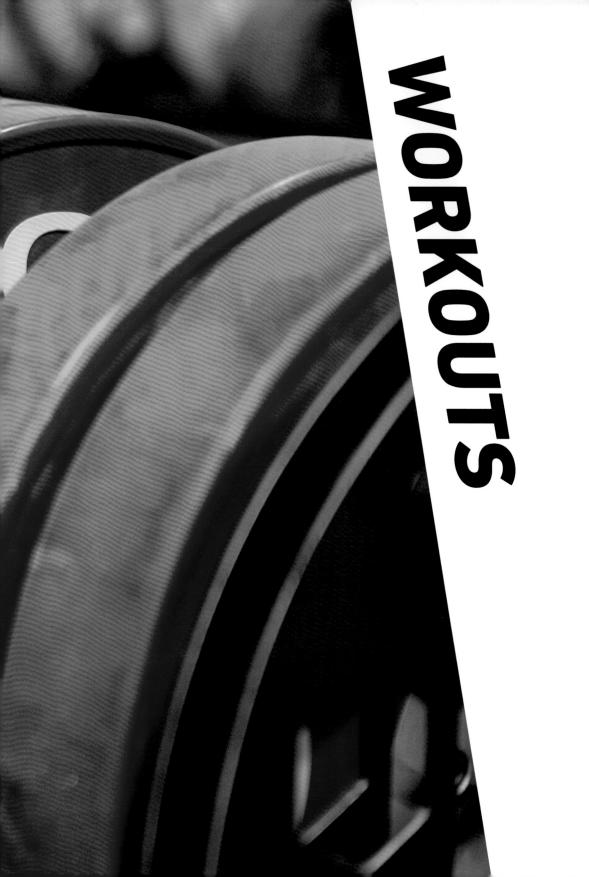

WORKOUTS

CREATING A TRAINING PROGRAM

If you truly want to sculpt your physique like a bodybuilder, you need to make a plan that will match your goals. There are three key steps to follow for creating your personalized training program.

[1] DEFINE YOUR TRAINING GOALS

The first step in developing your personalized training program is to clearly define your top three training goals. Begin by asking yourself some key questions:

- Is your goal to bulk up and add muscle mass, maintain existing muscle, or lean down and add definition?
- Do you want to train your entire body, or just specific muscle groups? Which three muscle groups are most important to you?
- Of the three goals, which is most important?
- Do your goals align with each other, and not conflict?
- What is your timeframe for meeting these goals?

By establishing your goals, committing them to paper, and organizing them in order of importance, you've taken the first step in developing your program, and you can move to planning your training and prioritizing workouts. If your goal is to target specific muscle groups, you can structure your workouts so that your top three muscle groups come at the beginning of the week, when you're most fresh. Taking these small but critical steps will help you develop a plan and help you decide how to structure your workouts *before* you enter the gym.

Also, it's important to ensure your goals align and don't conflict with each other. Training itself is challenging, so don't make it harder by trying to accomplish goals that don't align. You'll find it tough to gain muscle if you're simultaneously training for a marathon!

[2] DECIDE ON A TRAINING SPLIT

Your training frequency, or "split," is simply the total number of days you opt to train each week, and it's the most important component of adhering to a plan.

An effective workout split should range from 4 to 6 days, with each day focused on a different muscle group, or with the type of movement changing between each training day. If you're just starting out, you should opt for a four-day split to start; you'll recover faster and get accustomed to lifting weights. If you're a seasoned lifter you may want to opt for a five- or six-day split, but if you can only train four days per week, you can still make the most of each training day by pushing heavier weight, keeping rest between sets to a minimum, and opting for tougher exercise variations.

As you begin to think about your split, be realistic and be honest with yourself. Think about how often you *can* train—not how often you *want* to train. You'll miss fewer training sessions, make better progress, and will be less apt to experience burnout or disappointment. And by creating a focused split that aligns with your goals and also fits into your lifestyle, you'll be able to plan your workouts in advance, while still giving your muscles sufficient time to recover between training sessions. Whatever you do choose for your split, remember that it's critical to rest between sets and to allow 48 to 72 hours of recovery between training the same muscle groups. Building in sufficient time for your muscles to rest and recover is just as important as spending time in the gym.

[3] CHOOSE A TRAINING STRATEGY

Each workout in this book includes suggested rep ranges and between-set recovery times for building muscle, maintaining muscle, or leaning down. If your goals vary for different muscle groups, you can adjust sets, reps, and pace on training days to make adjustments for particular areas of focus.

BUILD
(FOR GAINING MUSCLE MASS)

Sets and reps: You should perform 4 to 5 sets of 8 to 10 reps per workout, using heavy weights that are challenging, particularly for the last 2 to 3 reps of a set. Go heavy on big compound lifts, and include enough overall volume to stimulate your muscles to grow.

Cardio and finishers: For a traditional bulk, exclude cardio and just put all of your excess calories toward weight training. For a clean bulk (adding muscle while still cutting fat), cardio and finishers will help burn fat while you're still building muscle.

Rest and recovery: Include 1 to 3 minutes of rest between sets. Big, heavy compound lifts will require more recovery and about 2 to 3 minutes of rest between sets. Isolation exercises should be closer to 1 to 1-1/2 minutes of rest between sets, since they tend to be less taxing than compound movements.

MAINTAIN
(FOR MAINTAINING EXISTING MUSCLE MASS, OR MAINTAINING MUSCLE WHILE LEANING DOWN)

Sets and reps: You'll work your muscles hard, but with a bit less volume by performing 3 to 4 sets of 8 to 15 reps per workout, which will give you enough volume to keep hard-earned muscle. You should still go heavy on the compound lifts, as this can further help with maintaining hard-earned muscle.

Cardio and finishers: Including cardio and finishers in workouts is important to help maintain muscle and keep you lean.

Rest and recovery: Recovery between sets for maintaining muscle should be between 1 to 1-1/2 minutes, but if you're looking to maintain muscle while leaning down there should be less than 1 minute of rest between sets to ensure greater fat loss and to reap the fat-burning benefits of any cardio.

LEAN
(FOR CUTTING FAT AND ADDING DEFINITION)

Sets and reps: Sets should be in the range of 3 to 4, with 12 to 20 reps per workout. The combination of two or more exercises in the form of supersets and circuits will help you get additional cardio benefits. You can still go heavy on big compound lifts, but supersets and circuits should be kept lighter to help maintain a quick tempo.

Cardio and finishers: Including nontraditional cardio and finishers is essential for successful leaning. If you're struggling to complete the nontraditional cardio portion of your workouts, you can replace 20 minutes of nontraditional cardio with 20 minutes of steady-state cardio at the end of the existing cardio workouts.

Rest and recovery: Recovery between sets for a leaning program should be short, between 30 and 45 seconds.

GOAL	SETS	REPS	WEIGHT	REST BETWEEN SETS
BUILD	4–5	8–10	HEAVY	1:00–3:00
MAINTAIN	3–4	8–15	HEAVY/MODERATE	1:00–1:30
MAINTAIN/LEAN	3–4	8–15	HEAVY/MODERATE	:45–1:00
LEAN	3–4	12–20	MODERATE	:30–:45

4 DAY SPECIALIZED WORKOUT

If you only have four days to devote to training, this plan will help you maximize your time, get leaner, and improve the details of your physique. This specialized split allows for more emphasis on aesthetics, with HIIT circuits and finishers included on the upper body days.

	DAY 1	DAY 2	DAY 3	DAY 4
				SPLIT
	BACK/BICEPS/ABS	**CHEST/TRICEPS**		**LEGS**
STRENGTH	T-bar row	Dumbbell incline bench press		Landmine squat
	Close-grip lat pulldown	Incline cable flye		Straight-leg deadlift
	Dumbbell pullover	Cross-body chest press		Barbell hack squat
	Bent-over barbell row	Close-grip bench press		Glute bridge
	EZ bar drag curl	Between-benches dips		Standing calf raise
	Spider curl	Skullcrushers	REST	**Superset:** Seated leg curl and leg extension
	Inverted row	Triceps pushdown		Seated calf raise
CARDIO & FINISHERS	**ABS CIRCUIT:** medicine ball slams 2x10; vacuum 3x15 seconds; reverse crunch 3x20; flutter kicks 3x30 seconds	**HIIT TREADMILL CIRCUIT:** 10% incline, 5x20 seconds all out sprint (rest 2-4 minutes between sprints)		

Exercises

Barbell hack squat (p.68)
Bent-over barbell row (p.98)
Burpee (p.176)
Close-grip bench press (p.128)
Close-grip lat pulldown (p.94)
Cross-body chest press (p.118)
Dumbbell incline bench press (p.116)
Dumbbell pullover (p.108)

EZ-bar drag curl (p.135
Flutter kicks (p.167)
Glute bridge (p.76)
High knees (p.178)
Incline bench cable high row (p.148)
Incline cable flye (p.122)
Inverted row (p.110)
Knee-ups (p.164)
Landmine squat (p.62)
Lateral raise (p.152)
Leg extension (p.88)

Medicine ball slams (p.160)
Military press (p.144)
Plank (p.166)
Reverse crunch (p.172)
Reverse flye (p.154)
Russian twist (p.170)
Seated calf raise (p.84)
Seated leg curl (p.80)
Skullcrushers (p.138)
Speed skater (p.179)
Spider curl (p.136)
Standing calf raise (p.82)

Straight-leg deadlift (p.72)
Switch lunge (p.181)
T-bar row (p.100)
Triceps pushdown (p.140)
Vacuum (p.161)
Wide-grip upright row (p.146)

Variations

Between-benches dips (p.125)
EZ bar partial-rep curl (p.133)
Narrow-to-wide press (p.145)
Side raises (p.165)

	DAY 5	DAY 6	DAY 7	SETS X REPS		
				BUILD	MAINTAIN	LEAN
	SHOULDERS/ABS					
	Military press (machine or barbell)			5x8	5x8	4x10
	Incline bench cable high row			5x8	5x8	4x10
	Narrow-to-wide press			5x8	4x8	3x15
	Lateral raise			5x8	4x10	3x15
	Reverse flye			4x10	4x10	3x15
	Wide-grip upright row			4x10	4x8	3x15
	EZ bar partial-rep curl			4xAMRAP	4xAMRAP	4xAMRAP
	TABATA CIRCUIT (2X): burpee; high knees; speed skater; switch lunge **ABS CIRCUIT (2X30 REPS):** knee-ups; side raises; Russian twist; plank	REST	REST			

NOTES

- Perform full sets for each exercise in the supersets
- Between-set rest (build): 2 minutes
- Between-set rest (maintain): 1 minute
- Between-set rest (lean): 30–45 seconds

4 DAY PUSH-PULL WORKOUT

This workout features combinations of pushing and pulling exercises to work muscle groups more efficiently. Opposing muscle groups are worked mostly with supersets, and hitting the legs twice during the week means more frequency, which is good for overall growth as well as leaning.

	SPLIT			
	DAY 1	**DAY 2**	**DAY 3**	**DAY 4**
	BACK/CHEST/ABS	LEGS		SHOULDERS/ARMS
STRENGTH	Bent-over barbell row	Sumo squat		Military press (with mid-rep pause)
	Superset: dumbbell incline bench press and high incline supine row			Wide-grip upright row
	Superset: dumbbell bench press and dumbbell upright row	**Superset:** goblet squat and straight-leg dumbbell deadlift		**Giant set:** neutral-grip dumbbell press; hammer curl; bench dips
	Superset: close-grip lat pulldown and decline push-up	**Superset:** Nordic curl and leg extension	REST	**Giant Set:** incline bench flye; incline bench skullcrushers; EZ bar drag curl
	Superset: bench dips and inverted row	**Superset:** single-leg glute bridge and standing calf raise		**Superset:** kickbacks and seated dumbbell curl
	Close-grip lat pulldown (1x50 reps at 40-50% weight)	Seated calf raise (partials: 7 at the top, 7 at the bottom, and 7 full reps)		
				Decline push-up
CARDIO & FINISHERS	**Abs circuit:** medicine ball slams 2x10; oblique throws 2x10 per side; plank 2x30 seconds; side plank 1x30 seconds per side	**Circuit:** 1x10 reps each: dynamic step-ups, line jumps, bench popovers, pop squat		**Stationary bike ladder sprints:** 30 sec/30 sec/25 sec/25 sec/20 sec/20 sec (ride 2–4 minutes between sprints, then cool down)

Exercises

Bench dips (p.130)
Bench popovers (p.186)
Bent-over barbell row (p.98)
Bulgarian split squat (p.66)
Cable pull-through (p.74)
Close-grip lat pulldown (p.94)
Decline push-up (p.120)
Dumbbell incline bench press (p.116)
Dynamic step-ups (p.183)
EZ bar drag curl (p.135)
Inverted row (p.110)

Leg extension (p.88)
Line jumps (p.185)
Medicine ball slams (p.160)
Military press (p.144)
Nordic curl (p.78)
Plank (p.166)
Pop squat (p.182)
Quad step-up (p.70)
Seated calf raise (p.84)
Standing calf raise (p.82)
Wide-grip upright row (p.146)
Zercher squat (p.64)

Variations

Dumbbell bench press (p.115)
Dumbbell single-leg calf raise (p.83)
Dumbbell upright row (p.147)
Front squat (p.61)
Goblet squat (p.61)
Hammer curl (p.133)
High incline supine row (p.103)
Incline bench flye (p.123)
Incline bench skullcrushers (p.139)

Kickbacks (p.141)
Neutral-grip dumbbell press (p.145)
Oblique throws (p.160)
Reverse lunge (p.87)
Seated dumbbell curl (p.133)
Side plank (p.166)
Single-leg glute bridge (p.77)
Straight-leg dumbbell deadlift (p.73)
Sumo squat (p.61)

DAY 5	DAY 6	DAY 7	SETS X REPS		
LEGS			BUILD	MAINTAIN	LEAN
Front squat			5x8	5x8	4x10
Superset: straight-leg dumbbell deadlift and Zercher squat			5x8	4x10	4x10
Superset: quad step-up and Bulgarian split squat			4x10	4x8	3x15
Superset: dumbbell single-leg calf raise and cable pull-through			4x10	4x8	3x15
Superset: seated calf raise and reverse lunge	REST	REST	4x10	4x8	3x15
			3xAMRAP	2xAMRAP	4xAMRAP

NOTES

- Perform full sets for each exercise in the supersets and giant sets
- Between-set rest (build): 2 minutes
- Between-set rest (maintain): 1 minute
- Between-set rest (lean): 30–45 seconds

4 DAY UPPER-LOWER WORKOUT

This workout features less specialization and more compound movements to make it particularly good for leaning down or plateau busting.
The compound movements are done first, followed by isolation exercises, and cardio and finishers are included on the upper body days.

		SPLIT		
	DAY 1	**DAY 2**	**DAY 3**	**DAY 4**
	LOWER BODY/ABS	**CHEST/BACK/BICEPS**		**LOWER BODY/ABS**
STRENGTH	Squat	High incline bench press		**Superset:** landmine squat and straight-leg deadlift
	Straight-leg dumbbell deadlift	High incline supine row		**Superset:** Smith machine Zercher squat and Smith machine glute bridge
	Sumo squat	Machine military press		**Superset:** seated calf raise and walking lunge
	Glute bridge	**Superset:** Incline cable flye and reverse cable flye		**Superset:** heel-elevated dumbbell hack squat and goblet squat
	Superset: high-box step-up and Nordic curl	**Superset:** cross-bench pullover and single-arm bent-over row	**REST**	
	Giant set: seated leg curl; leg extension; seated calf raise	Hammer curl		
		Close-grip EZ bar press		
CARDIO & FINISHERS	**ABS CIRCUIT:** cable chop 2x15; cable chop (low to high) 2x15; reverse crunch 3x20; flutter kicks 2x30 seconds	**ROWER:** 5x250m all out (2–4 minutes recovery between sprints)		**ABS CIRCUIT:** medicine ball slams 2x10; oblique throws 2x10 each side; plank 3x30 seconds; vacuum 3x15 seconds

Exercises

Burpee (p.176)
Cable chop (p.162)
Decline push-up (p.120)
Dynamic step-ups (p.183)
Flutter kicks (p.167)
Glute bridge (p.76)
High knees (p.178)
High row (p.150)
Incline cable flye (p.122)
Landmine squat (p.62)
Leg extension (p.88)
Medicine ball slams (p.160)
Nordic curl (p.78)

Plank (p.166)
Pop squat (p.182)
Reverse crunch (p.172)
Seated calf raise (p.84)
Seated leg curl (p.80)
Speed skater (p.179)
Spider curl (p.136)
Squat (p.60)
Straight-leg deadlift (p.72)
Switch lunge (p.181)
Vacuum (p.161)

Variations

Close-grip EZ bar press (p.129)
Cross-bench pullover (p.109)
Dumbbell bench press (p.115)
Dumbbell upright row (p.147)
EZ bar partial-rep curl (p.133)
Goblet squat (p.61)
Hammer curl (p.133)

Heel-elevated dumbbell hack squat (p.69)
High-box step-up (p.71)
High incline bench press (p.117)
High incline supine row (p.103)
Kickbacks (p.141)
Low-pulley cable row (p.105)
Machine military press (p.144)
Narrow-to-wide press (p.145)

Oblique throws (p.161)
Reverse cable flye (p.155)
Single-arm bent-over row (p.99)
Smith machine glute bridge (p.77)
Smith machine Zercher squat (p.65)
Straight-leg dumbbell deadlift (p.73)
Sumo squat (p.61)
Walking lunge (p.87)

	DAY 5	DAY 6	DAY 7	SETS X REPS		
				BUILD	MAINTAIN	LEAN
	SHOULDERS/UPPER BACK/TRICEPS					
	Dumbbell bench press			5x8	4x10	4x10
	Dumbbell upright row			5x8	4x10	4x10
	Narrow-to-wide press	REST	REST	4x10	4x8	3x15
	Low-pulley cable row			4x10	4x8	3x15
	Superset: high row and kickbacks			4x10	4x8	3x15
	Superset: decline push-up and spider curl			4x8	3x10	3x12
	EZ bar partial-rep curl			3xAMRAP	4xAMRAP	4xAMRAP
	BODYWEIGHT CIRCUIT: 4x2 min. 30 sec. on/30 sec. rest between exercises. 2 min. rest between sets. Choose four: burpee, high knees, switch lunge, dynamic step-ups, speed skater, pop squat			**NOTES** • Perform full sets for each exercise in the supersets and giant sets • Between-set rest (build): 2 minutes • Between-set rest (maintain): 1 minute • Between-set rest (lean): 30–45 seconds		

5 DAY PUSH-PULL WORKOUT

This workout features increased frequency, which helps accelerate muscle growth. Supersets allow for more volume and greater calorie burn, and post-workout cardio and finishers help with leaning.

				SPLIT
	DAY 1	**DAY 2**	**DAY 3**	**DAY 4**
	LEGS/ABS	BACK/CHEST	BICEPS/TRICEPS/ABS	LEGS
STRENGTH	**Superset:** landmine squat and landmine straight-leg deadlift	**Superset:** single-arm bent-over row and bench press	**Superset:** bench dips and hammer curl (seated)	**Superset:** Zercher split squat and straight-leg deadlift
	Superset: quad step-up and straight-leg deadlift	**Superset:** close-grip lat pulldown and decline push-up	**Superset:** skullcrushers and EZ bar drag curl	**Superset:** sumo squat and dumbbell single-leg calf raise
	Superset: seated calf raise and leg extension	**Superset:** T-bar row and incline cable flye	**Superset:** straight bar pushdown and spider curl	**Superset:** standing calf raise and reverse lunge
	Superset: Nordic curl and heel-elevated dumbbell hack squat	**Superset:** straight-arm pushdown and decline cable flye	**Superset:** kickbacks and standing biceps curl (alternating arms)	**Superset:** seated leg curl and leg extension
	Superset: goblet squat and cable pull-through	**Superset:** inverted row and pike push-up		Walking lunge
CARDIO & FINISHERS	**ABS CIRCUIT (3X):** vacuum 15 sec; tuck-up, x30; plank 30 seconds; reverse crunch x30		**SPIN BIKE SPRINT LADDER:** 25 sec/20 sec/15 sec/20 sec/ 25 sec (rest 2–5 minutes between each sprint) **ABS CIRCUIT (3X):** scissor kicks 30 sec; flutter kicks 30 sec; side plank 30 seconds each side; Russian twist x30	

Exercises

Bench dips (p.130)
Bench press (p.114)
Burpee (p.176)
Cable pull-through (p.74)
Cable row (p.104)
Close-grip lat pulldown (p.94)
Decline push-up (p.120)
Dumbbell pullover (p.108)
EZ bar drag curl (p.135)
Flutter kicks (p.167)
Front raise (p.156)
High knees (p.178)
Incline cable flye (p.122)
Inverted row (p.110)
Jumping jack (p.180)

Landmine squat (p.62)
Lateral raise (p.152)
Leg extension (p.88)
Military press (p.144)
Plank (p.166)
Nordic curl (p.78)
Quad step-up (p.70)
Reverse crunch (p.172)
Russian twist (p.170)
Seated calf raise (p.84)
Seated leg curl (p.80)
Skullcrushers (p.138)
Spider curl (p.136)
Standing biceps curl (p.132)
Standing calf raise (p.82)
Straight-leg deadlift (p.72)

Supine dumbbell row (p.102)
Switch lunge (p.181)
T-bar row (p.100)
Vacuum (p.161)

Variations

Decline cable flye (p.123)
Dumbbell single-leg calf raise (p.83)
Goblet squat (p.61)
Hammer curl (p.133)
Heel-elevated dumbbell hack squat (p.69)
High-row with external rotation (p.150)
Kickbacks (p.141)
Landmine straight-leg deadlift (p.73)
Neutral-grip dumbbell press (p.145)
Pike push-up (p.121)
Reverse lunge (p.87)

Scissor kicks (p.167)
Side plank (p.166)
Single-arm bent-over row (p.99)
Straight bar pushdown (p.141)
Straight-arm pushdown (p.109)
Sumo squat (p.61)
Tuck-up (p.169)
Walking lunge (p.87)
Wide-grip lat pulldown (p.95)
Zercher split squat (p.65)

	DAY 5	DAY 6	DAY 7	SETS X REPS		
	SHOULDERS/BACK			BUILD	MAINTAIN	LEAN
	Superset: supine dumbbell row and military press			5x8	4x10	4x10
	Superset: cable row and lateral raise			4x10	4x10	3x15
	Superset: dumbbell pullover and front raise			4x12	4x10	3x15
	Superset: wide-grip lat pulldown and neutral-grip dumbbell press			4x10	3x12	3x15
	High row with external rotation	REST	REST	3x15	3x12	3x10
	TABATA CIRCUIT 1: alternating burpees and jumping jacks (rest 2–4 minutes before starting circuit 2) **TABATA CIRCUIT 2:** alternating high-knees and switch lunges					

NOTES
- Perform full sets for each exercise in the supersets and giant sets
- Between-set rest (build): 2 minutes
- Between-set rest (maintain): 1 minute
- Between-set rest (lean): 30–45 seconds

5 DAY SPECIALIZED WORKOUT

This specialized split features increased volume to facilitate muscle growth, with more of an aesthetic emphasis on legs and shoulders to help develop the X-frame. Pay extra attention to time under tension to enhance the mind-muscle connection.

			SPLIT	
	DAY 1	DAY 2	DAY 3	DAY 4
	LEGS	SHOULDER/ABS	BACK/BICEPS/ABS	LEGS (DETAIL)
STRENGTH	Squat	Machine military press	Rack pull	**Superset:** split-stance landmine squat and landmine straight-leg deadlift
	Straight-leg deadlift	Lateral raise	Cable row	Single-leg glute bridge
	Heel-elevated dumbbell hack squat	Incline bench cable high row	Close-grip lat pulldown	Seated calf raise
	Glute bridge	**Superset:** neutral-grip dumbbell press and dumbbell upright row	Single-arm t-bar row	Leg extension
	Standing calf raise	Narrow-to-wide press	**Superset:** straight bar pushdown and dumbbell drag curl	Seated leg curl
	Lunge (2xAMRAP)	Seated EZ bar partial front raise	Hammer curl	Cable pull-through
CARDIO & FINISHERS		**ABS CIRCUIT:** scissor kicks 3x30; tuck-up 2x30; reverse crunch 2x30; plank 3x30 seconds; side plank 2x30 seconds (each side)	**HIIT:** max speed on stairclimber 6x30 seconds (rest 2-4 minutes between climbs)	**ABS CIRCUIT:** knee-ups 3x30; side raises 3x30 (each side); Russian twist 3x30; L-up 3x30

Exercises

Bench dips (p.130)
Cable pull-through (p.74)
Cable row (p.104)
Close-grip lat pulldown (p.94)
Cross-body chest press (p.118)
Glute bridge (p.76)
High knees (p.178)
Incline bench cable high row (p.148)
Jumping jack (p.180)
Knee-ups (p.164)

Lateral raise (p.152)
Leg extension (p.88)
Lunge (p.86)
Plank (p.166)
Rack pull (p.106)
Reverse crunch (p.172)
Russian twist (p.170)
Seated calf raise (p.84)
Seated leg curl (p.80)
Squat (p.60)
Standing calf raise (p.82)
Straight-leg deadlift (p.72)
Switch lunge (p.181)
Triceps pushdown (p.140)

Variations

Decline cable flye (p.123)
Dumbbell drag curl (p.135)
Dumbbell upright row (p.147)
Hammer curl (p.133)
Heel-elevated dumbbell hack squat (p.69)
High incline bench press (p.117)
High knees march (p.178)
Incline bench flye (p.123)
L-ups (p.165)
Landmine straight-leg deadlift (p.73)

Machine military press (p.145)
Narrow-to-wide press (p.145)
Neutral-grip dumbbell press (p.145)
Scissor kicks (p.167)
Seated EZ bar partial front raise (p.157)
Side plank (p.166)
Side raises (p.165)
Single-arm t-bar row (p.101)

Single-leg glute bridge (p.77)
Split-stance landmine squat (p.63)
Straight bar pushdown (p.141)
Tuck-up (p.169)
Weighted feet-elevated bench dips (p.131)

	DAY 5	DAY 6	DAY 7	SETS X REPS		
	CHEST/TRICEPS			**BUILD**	**MAINTAIN**	**LEAN**
	High incline bench press			4x10/8/8/6*	4x10/10/8/8*	4x10
	Incline bench flye			5x8	4x10	3x15
	Bench dips			4x10	3x12	3x15
	Superset: decline cable flye and triceps pushdown			4x12	4x10	3x12
	Cross-body chest press	REST	REST	4x12	4x8	3x15
	Weighted feet-elevated bench dips			3xAMRAP	3xAMRAP	3xAMRAP
	METABOLIC CIRCUIT: 4x2 minutes circuit of 30 seconds each: high knees, high knees march, jumping jack; switch lunge (rest 1-2 minutes between sets)			**NOTES** • (*) Reps decrease as sets progress • Perform full sets for each exercise in the the supersets • Between-set rest (build): 2 minutes • Between-set rest (maintain): 1 minute • Between-set rest (lean): 30–45 seconds		

5 DAY PUSH-PULL + LEGS WORKOUT

This workout is ideal for someone who wants to build their upper body while only maintaining legs. It's comprised mostly of straight and compound sets, and the training is split into movements, rather than by muscle groups. Cardio and finishers play a significant role in this workout.

		SPLIT		
	DAY 1	DAY 2	DAY 3	DAY 4
	PUSHING (SHOULDERS)	PULLING (VERTICAL)	LEGS	
STRENGTH	Military press	Close-grip lat pulldown	Front squat	
	Lateral raise	High incline supine row	Straight-leg deadlift	
	High incline bench press	**Superset:** single-arm pulldown with triceps pushdown	Zercher squat	
	Superset: incline bench flye and front raise	**Superset:** wide-grip lat pulldown and wide-grip upright row	**Superset:** high box step-up and cable pull-through	REST
	Superset: narrow-to-wide shoulder press and pike push-up	**Superset:** dumbbell partial pull and single-arm high row (chest-height)	**Superset:** standing calf raise and seated leg curl	
	Superset: triceps pushdown and kickbacks		**Superset:** leg extension and seated calf raise	
CARDIO & FINISHERS	**ABS CIRCUIT (2X):** medicine ball slams x10; plank 30 seconds; flutter kicks x30; reverse crunch x30	**HIIT:** treadmill sprints 6x15 seconds all-out at 10% incline (rest 2–4 minutes between sprints)		

Exercises

Bench dips (p.130)
Burpee (p.176)
Cable pull-through (p.74)
Close-grip lat pulldown (p.94)
Cross-body chest press (p.118)
Dumbbell pullover (p.108)
EZ bar drag curl (p.135)
Flutter kicks (p.167)
Front raise (p.156)
High row (p.150)
Jumping jack (p.180)
Knee-ups (p.164)

Lateral raise (p.152)
Leg extension (p.88)
Medicine ball slams (p.160)
Military press (p.144)
Plank (p.166)
Reverse crunch (p.172)
Russian twist (p.170)
Seated calf raise (p.84)
Seated leg curl (p.80)
Spider curl (p.136)
Standing biceps curl (p.132)
Standing calf raise (p.82)
Straight-leg deadlift (p.72)
Switch lunge (p.181)

T-bar row (p.100)
Triceps pushdown (p.140)
Wide-grip upright row (p.145)
Zercher squat (p.64)

Variations

Barbell incline bench press (p.117)
Dumbbell partial pull (p.107)
Flat bench flye (p.123)
Front squat (p.61)
High box step-up (p.71)
High incline bench press (p.117)
High incline supine row (p.103)
Incline bench flye (p.123)
Kickbacks (p.141)
Low-pulley cable row (p.105)

Narrow-to-wide press (p.145)
Neutral-grip dumbbell press (p.145)
Pike push-up (p.121)
Reverse cable flye (p.155)
Scissor kicks (p.167)
Side raises (p.165)
Single-arm bent-over row (p.99)
Single-arm high row (p.149)
Single-arm pulldown (p.95)
Walking lunge (p.87)
Wide-grip lat pulldown (p.95)

	DAY 5	DAY 6	DAY 7	SETS X REPS		
	PUSHING (CHEST)	**PULLING (HORIZONTAL)**		**BUILD**	**MAINTAIN**	**LEAN**
	Barbell incline bench press	T-bar row		5x8	4x10	3x15
	Neutral-grip dumbbell press	Low-pulley cable row		4x12	4x10	3x15
	Superset: cross-body chest press and lateral raise	**Superset:** dumbbell pullover and single-arm bent-over row		5x8	4x10	3x12
	Superset: flat bench flye and reverse cable flye	**Superset:** high row and EZ bar drag curl		4x12	4x10	3x12
	Superset: bench dips and kickbacks	**Superset:** high-incline supine row and spider curl	REST	4x10	4x8	3x12
	Triceps pushdown	Standing biceps curl (partial reps)		4x12	4x10	3x15
	HIIT FINISHER BODYWEIGHT CIRCUIT (2X): burpee 30 seconds; jumping jack 30 seconds; switch lunge 30 seconds; walking lunge x30 (rest 2 minutes between circuits)	**ABS CIRCUIT (2X):** knee-ups x30; side raises x20 each side; Russian twist 30 each side; scissor kicks 30 each side		**NOTES** • Perform full sets for each exercise in the supersets • Between-set rest (build): 2 minutes • Between-set rest (maintain): 1 minute • Between-set rest (lean): 30 to 45 seconds		

6 DAY SPECIALIZED WORKOUT

This split puts more emphasis on aesthetics, so you'll devote more time and attention to building and sculpting each muscle group, but the increased volume will still help promote muscle growth. Compound movements ensure that you train target muscles while still tying the entire physique together.

	DAY 1	DAY 2	DAY 3	DAY 4
SPLIT				
	LEGS	SHOULDERS	BACK/ABS	LEGS
STRENGTH	Barbell hack squat	Military press	T-bar row	Quad step-up
	Straight-leg deadlift	Wide-grip upright row	Wide-grip lat pulldown	Sumo squat
	Bulgarian split squat	Neutral-grip dumbbell press	Single-arm bent-over row	Standing calf raise
	Leg extension	Incline bench cable high row	Dumbbell pullover	**Superset:** front squat and split-stance landmine squat
	Superset: seated leg curl and dumbbell single-leg calf raise	Lateral raise	Single-arm pulldown	Glute bridge
		Reverse cable flye		**Superset:** heel-elevated dumbbell hack squat and Nordic curl
				Walking lunge
CARDIO & FINISHERS		**HIIT:** stationary/spin bike sprints 8x15 seconds all out (rest 2–4 minutes between sprints, or until heart rate drops to 60% of max)	**ABS CIRCUIT:** 2x30 reps each: plank, vacuum, V-up, Russian twist	

Exercises

Barbell hack squat (p.68)
Bench dips (p.130)
Bench press (p.114)
Bulgarian split squat (p.66)
Close-grip bench press (p.128)
Decline push-up (p.120)
Dips (p.124)
Dumbbell incline bench press (p.116)
Dumbbell pullover (p.108)
EZ bar drag curl (p.135)
Flutter kicks (p.167)
Glute bridge (p.76)

Incline bench cable high row (p.148)
Inverted row (p.110)
Lateral raise (p.152)
Leg extension (p.88)
Military press (p.144)
Nordic curl (p.78)
Plank (p.166)
Quad step-up (p.70)
Reverse crunch (p.172)
Russian twist (p.170)
Seated leg curl (p.80)
Single-arm pulldown (p.95)
Skullcrushers (p.138)

Standing biceps curl (p.132)
Standing calf raise (p.82)
Straight-leg deadlift (p.72)
T-bar row (p.100)
V-up (p.168)
Vacuum (p.161)
Wide-grip upright row (p.146)

Variations

Dumbbell single-leg calf raise (p.83)
EZ bar partial-rep curl (p.133)
Flat bench flye (p.123)
Front squat (p.61)
Heel-elevated dumbbell hack squat (p.69)
Incline bench flye (p.123)
Kickbacks (p.141)
Neutral-grip dumbbell press (p.145)
Reverse cable flye (p.155)
Side plank (p.166)

Single-arm bent-over row (p.99)
Sumo squat (p.61)
Split-stance landmine squat (p.63)
Walking lunge (p.87)
Wide-grip lat pulldown (p.95)

	DAY 5	DAY 6	DAY 7	SETS X REPS		
	CHEST	ARMS/ABS		BUILD	MAINTAIN	LEAN
	Dumbbell incline bench press	Bench dips		5x8	4x8	3x12
	Incline bench flye	Inverted row		5x8	4x10	3x15
	Dips	Skullcrushers		5x8	4x8	3x12
	Bench press	Standing biceps curl (alternating arms)		4x10	3x12	3x15
	Flat bench flye	Close-grip bench press		4x10	3x12	3x15
	Decline push-up	EZ bar drag curl		3xAMRAP	3xAMRAP	2xAMRAP
		Superset: EZ bar partial-rep curl (seated) and kickbacks	REST	3x20	3x20	3x20
	HIIT: rower 4x250m (rest 2–4 minutes between sprints, or until heart rate drops to 60% of max)	**ABS CIRCUIT:** 2x30 reps each: reverse crunch, flutter kicks, side plank, V-up				

NOTES

- Perform full sets for each exercise in the supersets and giant sets
- Between-set rest (build): 2 minutes
- Between-set rest (maintain): 1 minute
- Between-set rest (lean): 30–45 seconds

WORKOUT **8**

6 DAY PUSH-PULL + LEGS WORKOUT

The training in this workout is based on movements, rather than muscle splits, and the increased volume will help promote both muscle growth and fat loss. All related muscle groups will work in unison to create quick muscle growth while still maintaining aesthetics. You'll hit major muscle groups twice per week.

	SPLIT			
	DAY 1	**DAY 2**	**DAY 3**	**DAY 4**
	PUSH (VERTICAL)	**PULL (HORIZONTAL)**	**LEGS**	**PUSH (HORIZONTAL)**
STRENGTH	Military press	Rack pull	Landmine squat	Bench press
	Dumbbell bench press (high incline)	Cable upright row	Barbell hack squat	Bench press (low incline)
	Lateral raise	Single-arm t-bar row	**Superset:** Bulgarian split squat and quad step-up	Lateral raise
	Superset: neutral-grip dumbbell press and front raise	**Superset:** single-arm bent-over row and dumbbell pullover	**Superset:** leg extension and standing calf raise	**Superset:** cross-body chest press and triceps pushdown
	Superset: incline bench flye and reverse flye	**Superset:** high row and dumbbell drag curl	**Superset:** seated leg curl and seated calf raise	**Superset:** bench dips and kickbacks
	Superset: skullcrushers and close-grip EZ bar press	Spider curl	Cable pull-through	Skullcrushers (with EZ bar)
	Triceps pushdown	EZ bar partial-rep curl (seated)	Nordic curl	
CARDIO & FINISHERS		**HIIT:** stationary/spin bike 4x30 seconds all out, high tension (rest 2–4 minutes between sprints, or until heart rate drops to 60% of max)	**ABS CIRCUIT (3X):** vacuum 20 seconds; plank 40 seconds; L-ups x20; reverse crunch x30	

Exercises

Barbell hack squat (p.68)
Bench dips (p.130)
Bench press (p.114)
Bulgarian split squat (p.66)
Burpee (p.176)
Cable pull-through (p.74)
Close-grip lat pulldown (p.94)
Cross-body chest press (p.118)
Dumbbell pullover (p.108)
EZ bar drag curl (p.135)
Front raise (p.156)
Glute bridge (p.76)

High knees (p.178)
High row (p.150)
Landmine squat (p.62)
Lateral raise (p.152)
Leg extension (p.88)
Medicine ball slams (p.160)
Military press (p.144)
Nordic curl (p.78)
Plank (p.166)
Quad step-up (p.70)
Rack pull (p.106)
Reverse crunch (p.172)
Reverse flye (p.154)
Seated calf raise (p.84)

Seated leg curl (p.80)
Skullcrushers (p.138)
Spider curl (p.136)
Standing calf raise (p.82)
Supine dumbbell row (p.102)
Triceps pushdown (p.140)
V-up (p.168)
Vacuum (p.161)

Variations

Cable upright row (p.147)
Close-grip EZ bar press (p.129)
Dumbbell bench press (p.115)
Dumbbell drag curl (p.135)
EZ bar partial-rep curl (seated) (p.133)
Goblet squat (p.61)
Hammer curl (p.133)
Incline bench flye (p.123)
Kickbacks (p.141)
L-ups (p.165)

Landmine straight-leg deadlift (p.73)
Neutral-grip dumbbell press (p.145)
Oblique throws (p.160)
Single-arm bent-over row (p.99)
Single-arm cable row (p.105)
Single-arm pulldown (p.95)
Single-arm t-bar row (p.101)
Single-leg glute bridge (p.77)

Standing split squat (p.67)
Sumo squat (p.61)
Wide-grip lat pulldown (p.95)

	DAY 5	DAY 6	DAY 7	SETS X REPS		
	PULL (VERTICAL)	LEGS		BUILD	MAINTAIN	LEAN
	Wide-grip lat pulldown	Landmine straight-leg deadlift		5x8	4x10	4x10
	Cable upright row	Glute bridge		5x8	4x10	4x10
	Superset: single-arm pulldown and single-arm cable row (low pulley)	**Superset:** seated leg curl and standing split squat		5x8	4x10	3x12
	Superset: supine dumbbell row and spider curl	Sumo squat		5x8	4x10	3x15
	Superset: close-grip lat pulldown and EZ bar drag curl	**Superset:** standing calf raise and goblet squat	REST	4x10	3x15	3x15
	Hammer curl (seated)			4x10	3x15	3x15
		Single-leg glute bridge		AMRAP	AMRAP	AMRAP
	METABOLIC CIRCUIT: 5 minutes of 30 seconds on/30 seconds rest; choose between burpee and high knees	**ABS CIRCUIT (3X):** medicine ball slams x10; oblique throws x10 each side; V-up x 30 seconds		**NOTES** • Perform full sets for each exercise in the supersets • Between-set rest (build): 2 minutes • Between-set rest (maintain): 1 minute • Between-set rest (lean): 30–45 seconds		

6 DAY FREQUENCY + SPECIALIZATION WORKOUT

This specialized split emphasizes aesthetics, but the increased volume will still promote muscle growth. Abs circuits and HIIT finishers help complete this challenging workout!

				SPLIT
	DAY 1	**DAY 2**	**DAY 3**	**DAY 4**
	LEGS	**SHOULDERS**	**CHEST/BACK**	**LEGS**
STRENGTH	Squat	Military press	T-bar row	Walking lunge (3x20 reps)
	Quad step-up	Dumbbell upright row	Dumbbell incline bench press	**Superset:** barbell hack squat and straight-leg dumbbell deadlift
	Glute bridge	**Superset:** single-arm cable raise and high row with external rotation	**Superset:** wide-grip lat pulldown and decline push-up (pause mid-rep)	**Superset:** Bulgarian split squat and glute bridge
	Superset: cable pull-through and dumbbell single-leg calf raise	**Superset:** supine dumbbell row and reverse flye	**Superset:** single-arm cable row and incline cable flye	**Superset:** goblet squat and cable pull-through
	Superset: seated leg curl and leg extension	Narrow-to-wide press	**Superset:** single-arm pulldown and straight-bar pushdown	**Superset:** standing calf raise and leg extension
	Seated calf raise			
CARDIO & FINISHERS		**TABATA CIRCUIT (2X):** alternating speed skaters and pop squats (rest 2–3 minutes between circuits)	**ABS CIRCUIT (3X):** side plank 30 seconds each side; plank 30 seconds; vacuum 20 seconds	

Exercises

Barbell hack squat (p.68)
Bench dips (p.130)
Bulgarian split squat (p.66)
Cable pull-through (p.74)
Close-grip bench press (p.128)
Decline push-up (p.120)
Dips (p.124)
Dumbbell incline bench press (p.116)
Flutter kicks (p.167)
Front raise (p.156)
Glute bridge (p.76)
High row (p.150)

Incline cable flye (p.122)
Knee-ups (p.164)
Lateral raise (p.152)
Leg extension (p.88)
Military press (p.144)
Plank (p.166)
Pop squat (p.182)
Quad step-up (p.70)
Reverse crunch (p.172)
Reverse flye (p.154)
Russian twist (p.170)
Seated calf raise (p.84)
Seated leg curl (p.80)
Single-arm pulldown (p.96)

Speed skater (p.179)
Spider curl (p.136)
Squat (p.60)
Standing biceps curl (p.132)
Standing calf raise (p.82)
Supine dumbbell row (p.102)
T-bar row (p.100)
Vacuum (p.161)

Variations

Dumbbell drag curl (p.135)
Dumbbell single-leg calf raise (p.83)
Dumbbell upright row (p.147)
Feet-elevated inverted row (p.111)
Goblet squat (p.61)
High row with external rotation (p.150)
Incline bench skullcrushers (p.139)
Narrow-to-wide press (p.145)

Neutral-grip dumbbell press (p.145)
Seated EZ bar partial front raise (p.157)
Seated reverse flye (p.155)
Side plank (p.166)
Single-arm cable raise (p.153)
Single-arm cable row (p.105)
Straight-leg dumbbell deadlift (p.73)
Straight-bar pushdown (p.141)

Walking lunge (p.87)
Wide-grip lat pulldown (p.95)

DAY 5	DAY 6	DAY 7	SETS X REPS		
SHOULDERS	ARMS/CHEST/BACK		BUILD	MAINTAIN	LEAN
Superset: neutral-grip dumbbell press and dumbbell upright row	**Superset:** feet-elevated inverted row and decline push-up		5x8	4x10	4x10
Superset: lateral raise and seated reverse flye	Dips		4x10	4x8	4x8
Superset: narrow-to-wide press and front raise	Dumbbell drag curl		5x8	4x10	3x15
High row	**Superset:** close-grip bench press and standing biceps curl (alternating)	REST	4x10	3x15	3x12
	Superset: incline bench skullcrushers and spider curl		4x12	3x15	3x12
Seated EZ bar partial front raise	Bench dips		AMRAP	AMRAP	AMRAP
HIIT: rower 6x200m (rest 2–4 minutes between sets, or until heart rate drops to 60% of max)	**ABS CIRCUIT (3X30):** reverse crunch; flutter kicks; Russian twist, knee-ups		**NOTES** • Perform full sets for each exercise in the supersets and giant sets • Between-set rest (build): 2 minutes • Between-set rest (maintain): 1 minute • Between-set rest (lean): 30–45 seconds		

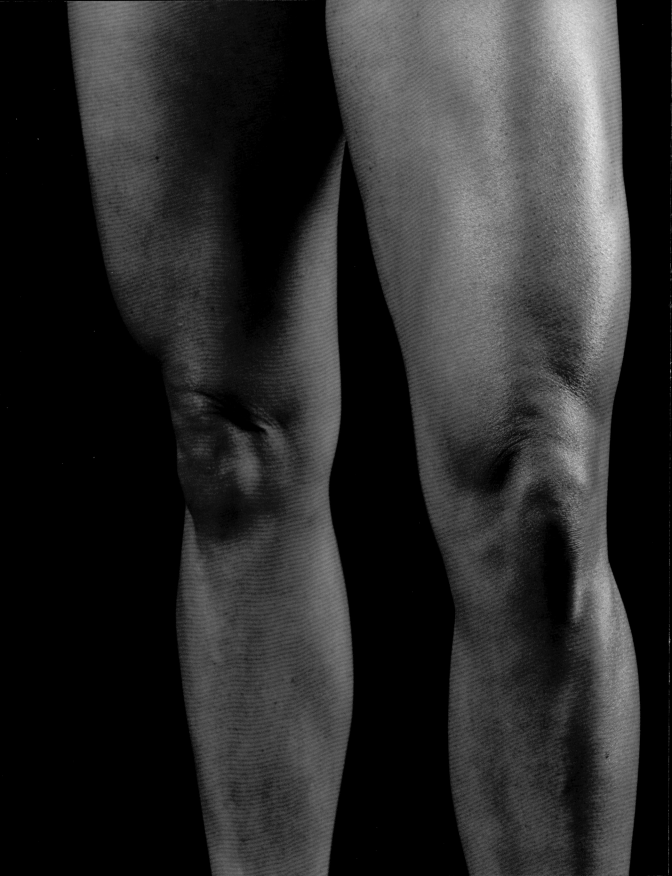

LEGS

TARGETS **///** quads, hamstrings, glutes (primary); calves, lower back (secondary)
EQUIPMENT **///** barbell, plates, squat or power rack

SQUAT

Often called the "king" of exercises, the squat helps sculpt the legs, increases overall muscle mass, improves overall strength, and boosts metabolism.

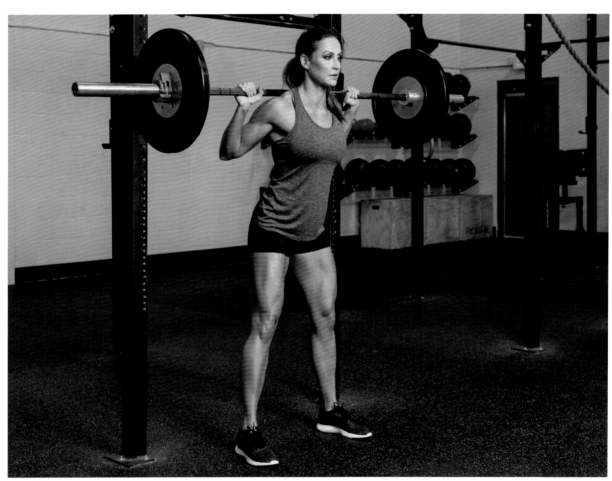

[1] Step under the bar, with your feet positioned slightly wider than shoulder-width apart. Place your hands on the bar, with your elbows pulled in and positioned directly under the bar. Place the bar on your traps and pin your shoulder blades back and against the bar. Take a deep breath and unrack the bar. Keeping your core tight and breathing normally, take a step forward with one foot, and then take a step forward with the other foot. (Imagine that your entire body is under a great tension—almost like a tight rubber band.) In preparation of the descent, take a deep breath and hold.

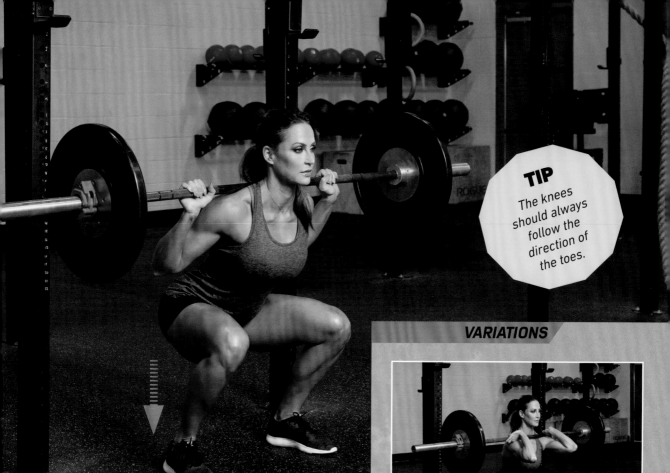

TIP
The knees should always follow the direction of the toes.

VARIATIONS

[2] Keeping your chest up, core tight, and weight pushed through your heels, sit back until your upper legs are parallel to the ground. Exhale as you push the weight back up, driving through your heels and focusing on pushing the weight with your legs.

Front squat (more challenging) The bar rests across the clavicle and in the divots of the shoulders. Hold the bar in a clean position and keep the elbows high and held out in front of you. (The quads are the focus with this variation.)

Sumo squat The bar placement is the same as the standard squat, but the stance is up to twice as wide, with the toes and knees pointed out. (Adductor and hamstrings are the focus with this variation.)

Goblet squat (easier) Hold a dumbbell perpendicular to the ground with palms under the top plate. Align your elbows directly under the dumbbell, with the top of the dumbbell almost touching your collarbone.

TRAIN THE RIGHT WAY

DO: start with lighter weight and slowly go through the full range of motion before attempting heavier weight.

DON'T: perform heavy squats if you aren't warmed up properly or have a history of back or knee problems.

TARGETS /// quads, glutes, hamstrings (primary); abs (secondary)
EQUIPMENT /// barbell and plates

LANDMINE SQUAT

This exercise builds muscle and strengthens the core, and helps keep pressure off the spine and knees. The bar provides stability and encourages proper form. If traditional squats are uncomfortable for you, this will be your new go-to.

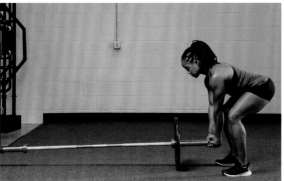

[1] Secure an Olympic bar in a sturdy corner or in a t-bar station. Place the plates on the bar. Stand at the end of the bar and position your feet shoulder-width apart. Clasp your hands under the end of the bar.

TIP

First try this with only the bar to help you get a feel for how to pick up and hold the weight, and also to get a sense of the range of motion.

[2] Lift the bar to your chest, and then cup your hands under the bar with the heels of your hands touching. Keep your elbows close and positioned directly underneath the bar. Step forward until the end of the bar is nearly resting on your collarbone.

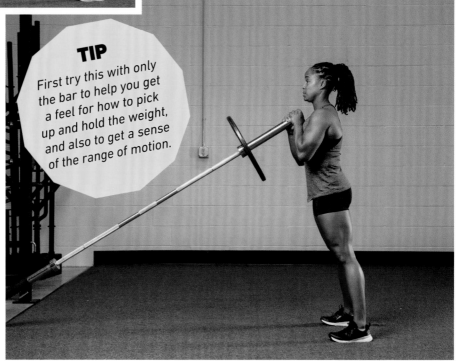

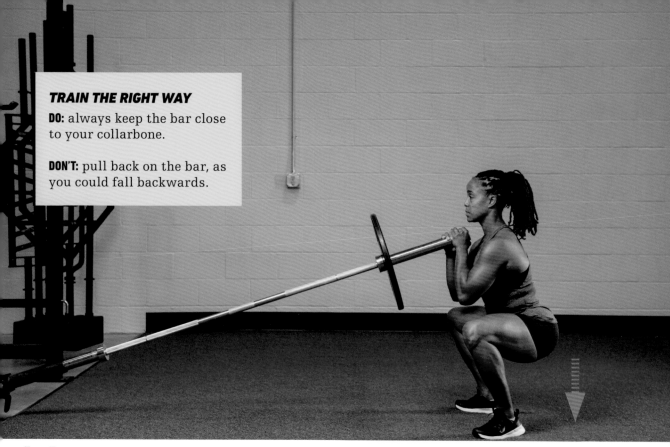

[3] Keeping your chest tall, press your weight slightly into the bar and allow the bar to guide your motion as you begin to squat. Pause when your upper legs are at parallel or just below.

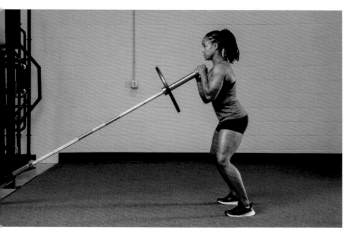

[4] Push through your legs to drive the bar back up to the starting position.

VARIATION

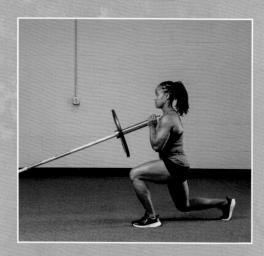

▲ **Split-stance landmine squat (more challenging)**
Grasp the end of the bar and place it near your collarbone. Take a small step forward with one leg and a step back with the other. Place equal weight on both legs and descend into a squat. (Perform all reps on one leg and then switch sides.)

TARGETS **///** quads, hamstrings, glutes (primary); core, biceps (secondary)
EQUIPMENT **///** barbell, plates, and squat or power rack

ZERCHER SQUAT

The unusual bar placement for this exercise helps targets the quads, hamstrings, glutes, and leg stabilizers to encourage proper form for the entire body. Perfect this lift and all other squat variations will be more effective!

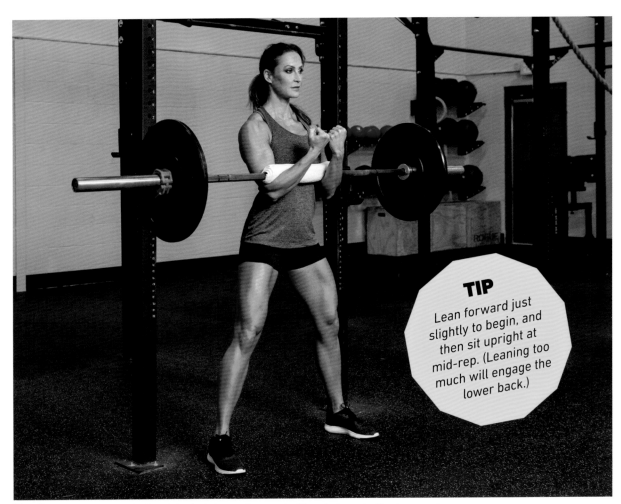

TIP

Lean forward just slightly to begin, and then sit upright at mid-rep. (Leaning too much will engage the lower back.)

[1] Position the barbell at hip-height on the rack. Stand close to the bar and place your arms under the bar, resting it in the bend of your elbows and just below the biceps. Unrack the bar and hold it close to your midsection, keeping your hands close together and your upper body tall.

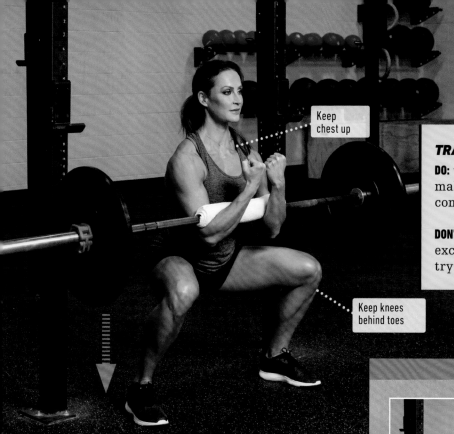

Keep chest up

Keep knees behind toes

TRAIN THE RIGHT WAY

DO: use a bar pad or towel to make the exercise more comfortable on your arms.

DON'T: load up the bar with excess weight before first trying this exercise.

VARIATIONS

[2] Engage your core, place your weight through your heels, and slowly squat. Pause momentarily when your upper legs reach parallel.

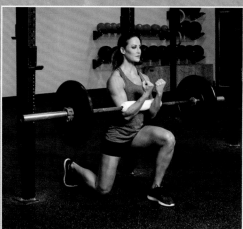

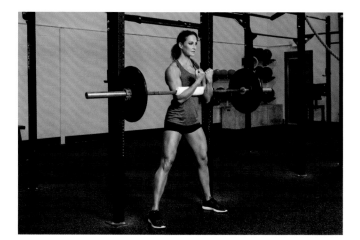

Zercher split squat (more challenging) Hold the bar in the crook of your arms and keep it close to your body. Stand in a lunge position, and slowly lower your body down until the front upper leg reaches parallel. Switch your stance and repeat on the opposite side.

Smith machine Zercher squat (easier) Set the bar to hip height on the Smith machine and perform the exercise as you would on the squat rack. (This variation can help beginners get a feel for the exercise. It's also beneficial for those who wish to go heavier on the lift.)

[3] Engage your quads, glutes, and hamstrings to drive the bar upward and bring your body back up into a standing position.

BULGARIAN SPLIT SQUAT

This unilateral exercise is excellent for building muscle in the legs, increasing overall strength, and improving balance. It also can balance out asymmetries and improve core strength, and since you're training one leg at a time, it's a great way to train heavy without putting excessive pressure on the back.

[1] Facing away from the bench, hold the dumbbells at your sides and place the toes of your dominant leg on the bench. Stand far enough from the bench that your rear lower leg is parallel to the ground.

TIP
Start with your non-dominant leg to determine the number of reps you do on your dominant leg.

Keep upper body tall throughout range of motion

VARIATION

[2] Lower your body until your front upper leg is parallel to the ground, and then push through your front heel to drive your body up and back into the starting position.

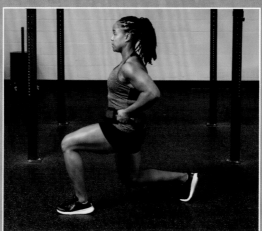

Standing split squat (easier) Hold a dumbbell in the same hand as your leading leg, stand in a lunge position, and lower your body until your front upper leg reaches parallel. Switch legs and repeat on the opposite side to complete one set.

TARGETS **///** quads, hamstrings, glutes (primary); calves, lower back (secondary)
EQUIPMENT **///** barbell and plates (bumper plates are ideal)

BARBELL HACK SQUAT

The barbell hack squat is a classic lift and one of the best compound exercises for quad development. If you're looking to build a beautiful quad sweep and gain strength and power, this should be your go-to leg exercise!

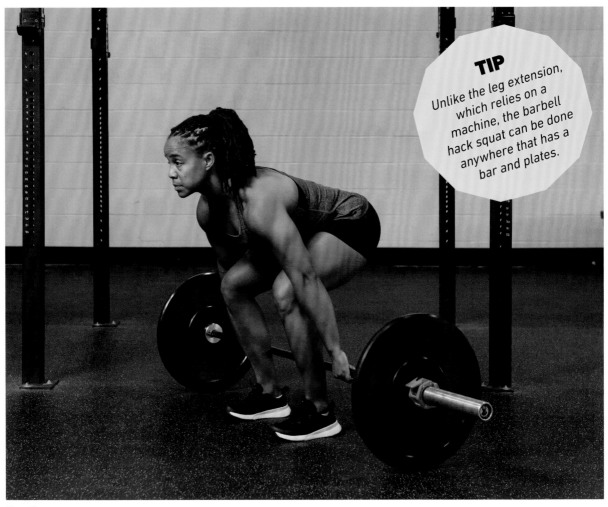

TIP
Unlike the leg extension, which relies on a machine, the barbell hack squat can be done anywhere that has a bar and plates.

[1] Begin with the bar placed behind your legs. Using squat form with your feet positioned shoulder-width apart and your toes pointing slightly outward, grasp the bar using an overhand grip with your hands placed slightly wider than your legs.

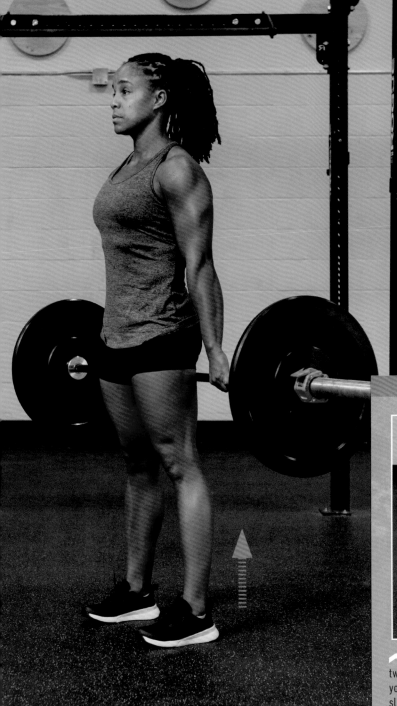

VARIATIONS

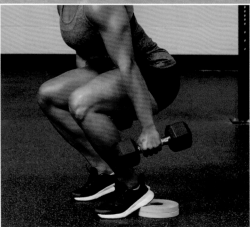

Heel-elevated dumbbell hack squat (easier) Place two small plates on the floor and shoulder-width apart. Place your heels on the plates. Hold dumbbells at your sides and slightly behind you, keeping your upper body tall and the dumbbells behind you throughout the range of motion.

Heel-elevated barbell hack squat (easier) Place two small plates shoulder-width apart and then place your heels on the plates. (This option is good if you're a beginner or lack the flexibility to go through a full range of motion.)

[2] With your shoulders back and chest up, slowly pull the bar up while pushing yourself into a standing position until your legs are fully extended. Slowly lower the bar back down to the starting position.

TARGETS /// quads (primary); hamstrings, glutes, calves (secondary)
EQUIPMENT /// dumbbells and standard bench

QUAD STEP-UP

By slowing down this exercise and pulling yourself up with your lead leg rather than pushing with your trail leg, you'll switch the focus from the posterior chain to the quads. The result will be a well-developed quad sweep and an improvement in overall balance and body awareness.

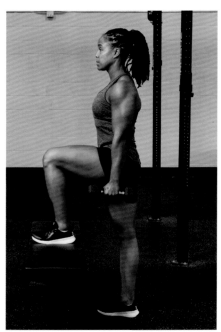

[1] Hold the dumbbells at your sides using a neutral grip. Stand facing a flat bench with one foot placed flat on the bench.

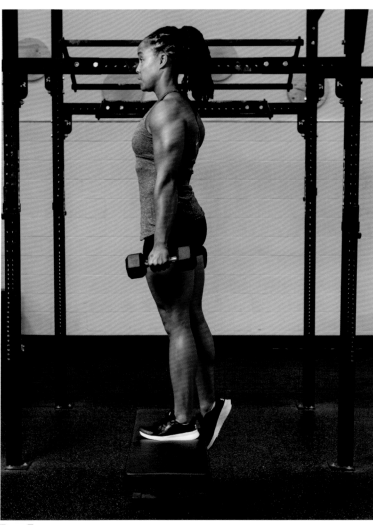

[2] Pull your body up to a standing position on top of the bench, while keeping your weight on your "pulling" leg.

TRAIN THE RIGHT WAY

DO: take your time going through each rep; don't rush.

DON'T: use momentum to get through the last few reps.

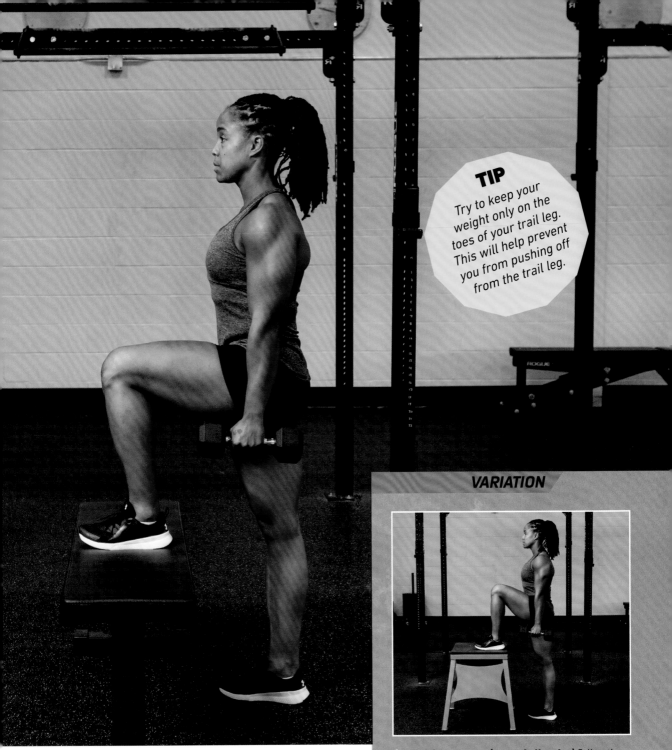

TIP
Try to keep your weight only on the toes of your trail leg. This will help prevent you from pushing off from the trail leg.

VARIATION

[3] Using the same leg, slowly step down from the bench. Repeat all reps on one leg before switching to the opposite leg.

⌃ **High box step-up (more challenging)** Follow the same steps, but use a tall plyo box or platform to hit both the quads and the glutes.

TARGETS /// hamstrings (primary); glutes, lower back (secondary)
EQUIPMENT /// barbell and plates

STRAIGHT-LEG DEADLIFT

Hamstrings are responsible for two important types of movement: knee flexion and hip extension. The straight-leg deadlift trains the hamstrings through a full hip extension to help improve strength, speed, and knee stability.

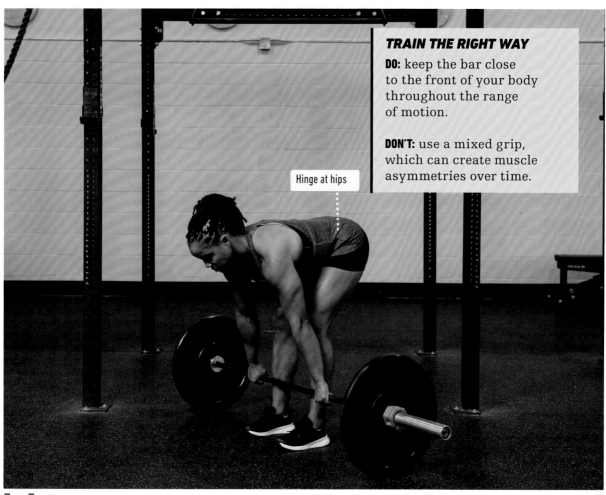

Hinge at hips

TRAIN THE RIGHT WAY

DO: keep the bar close to the front of your body throughout the range of motion.

DON'T: use a mixed grip, which can create muscle asymmetries over time.

[1] Stand behind the bar with your feet positioned shoulder-width apart. Bend at the hips and grasp the bar with an overhand grip that is slightly wider than shoulder-width apart.

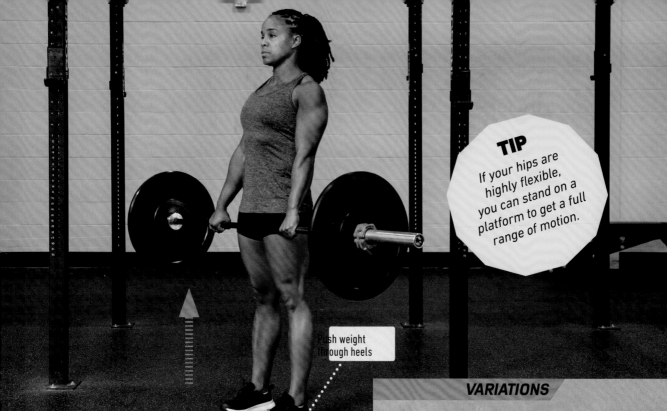

TIP
If your hips are highly flexible, you can stand on a platform to get a full range of motion.

Push weight through heels

[2] With a tight core and a flat back, slowly pull the weight up until you're standing tall. (Keep your legs straight, but don't lock your knees.)

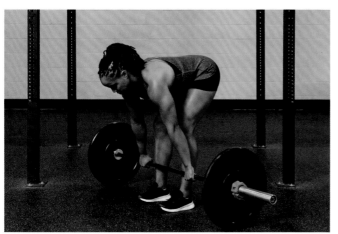

[3] Slowly lower the weight all the way back down to the starting position, or until you feel your back just starting to round.

VARIATIONS

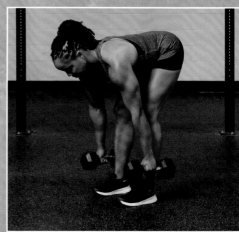

⌃ **Straight-leg dumbbell deadlift (easier)** Hold dumbbells either in front of you or at your sides. (Holding dumbbells at your sides can help target more glutes, while holding dumbbells in front will help target more hamstrings.)

Landmine straight-leg deadlift (more challenging) Place smaller plates on the bar to create more range of motion. Stand at the end of the bar and interlock your hands underneath it, with your feet shoulder-width apart, or slightly wider. Push into the bar as you stand up.

TARGETS /// glutes, hamstrings (primary); lower back (secondary)
EQUIPMENT /// low-pulley cable and rope attachment

CABLE PULL-THROUGH

The cable pull-through teaches better hip extension, which is critical for performing compound lifts and for kettlebell work. It's also great for developing the glutes and hamstrings. The cable provides constant tension, which helps improve the mind-muscle connection.

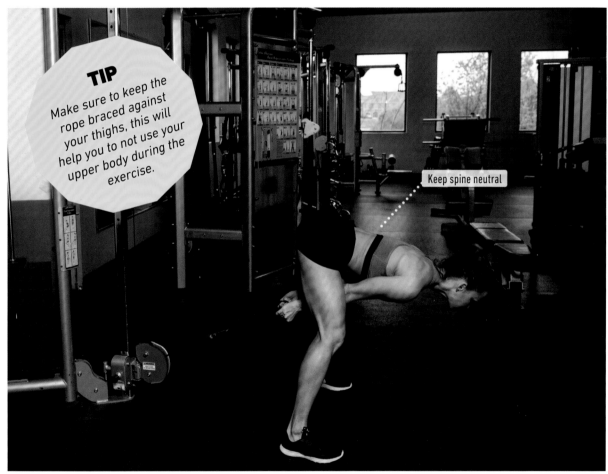

TIP
Make sure to keep the rope braced against your thighs, this will help you to not use your upper body during the exercise.

Keep spine neutral

[1] Set the cable to the lowest pin and attach the rope attachment. Face away from the cable and straddle the rope, reach down and grab the ends of the rope attachment with an overhand grip, and secure the rope against your inner thighs. Walk out about 2 to 3 feet (.5m to 1m), or until you feel tension in the cables. With your feet shoulder-width apart and soft knees, hinge at the hip and slowly lower your upper body down toward the ground.

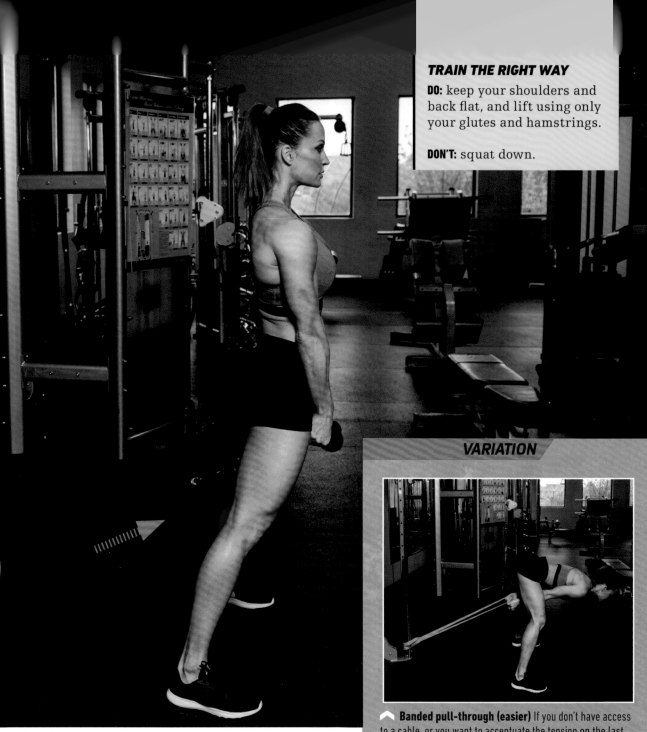

TRAIN THE RIGHT WAY

DO: keep your shoulders and back flat, and lift using only your glutes and hamstrings.

DON'T: squat down.

VARIATION

[2] Explosively push your hips forward while pulling the rope upward until you achieve a full hip extension (the movement of this exercise should very closely resemble a kettlebell swing).

▲ **Banded pull-through (easier)** If you don't have access to a cable, or you want to accentuate the tension on the last quarter of the rep, banded pull-throughs are the perfect alternative. Secure a resistance band to the bottom of a stable object, grasp the other end of the band with both hands, and perform the exercise as you would with cables.

TARGETS /// glutes, hamstrings (primary); lower back (secondary)
EQUIPMENT /// bar and 45lb bumper plates

GLUTE BRIDGE

The gluteus maximus is the largest muscle in the body, and well-developed glutes are not only attractive, they're powerful. Glute bridges are the best exercise for activating and sculpting the glutes, and strong glutes mean strong squats and deadlifts, as well as the ability to run faster and jump higher.

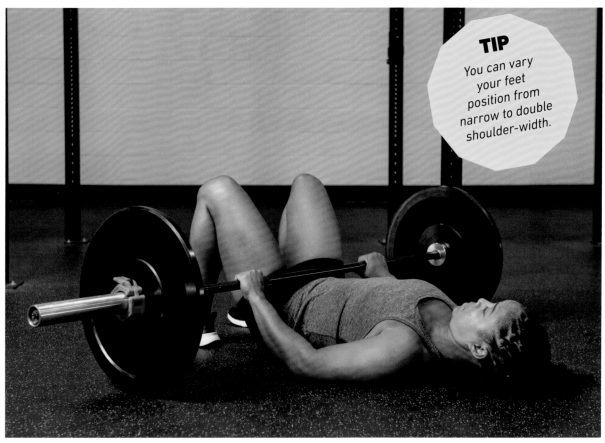

TIP
You can vary your feet position from narrow to double shoulder-width.

[1] Sit on the ground with your legs fully extended and toes pointed. Roll the bar up until it's resting directly over your hips. Lie back and pull your heels in as close to your glutes as possible. Brace your arms against the bar and tuck your chin to your chest.

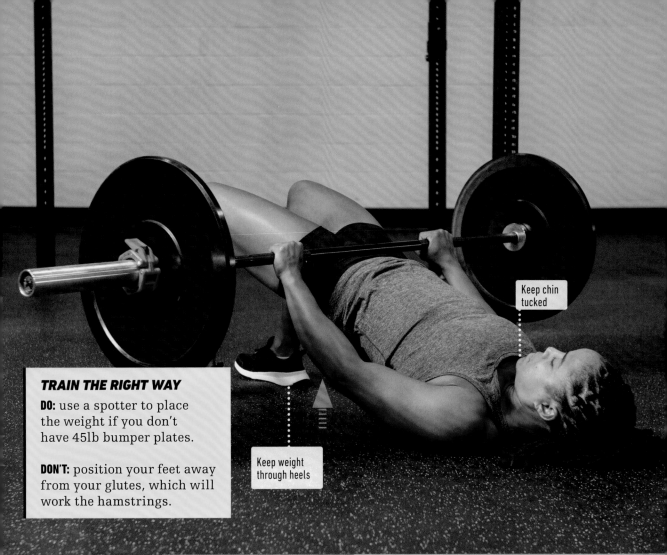

Keep chin
tucked

Keep weight
through heels

TRAIN THE RIGHT WAY

DO: use a spotter to place
the weight if you don't
have 45lb bumper plates.

DON'T: position your feet away
from your glutes, which will
work the hamstrings.

[2] Engage your
glutes and
push the bar upward
until you reach a full
hip extension, then
lower your hips back
down to just above
the ground.

VARIATIONS

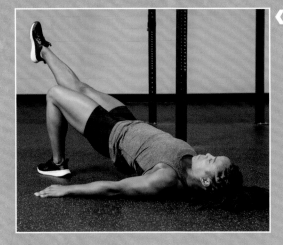

‹ Single-leg glute bridge (easier)
Lie flat on the ground with your feet
close to your glutes. Extend your
dominant leg straight out and push your
glutes upward with the opposite leg.
Keep your hips square to the ground and
keep your chin tucked. Repeat the
movement with the opposite leg.

Smith machine glute bridge (easier)
This version is good if you have a hard
time getting the weight over your hips.
Set the safety to allow you to get under
the bar and use a bar pad. The form is
the same as traditional glute bridges.

TARGETS /// hamstrings (primary); calves, glutes, lower back (secondary)
EQUIPMENT /// exercise mat

NORDIC CURL

This top exercise for strengthening the hamstrings requires only your bodyweight to execute. You'll help prevent injuries and build the perfect hamstring peak when you incorporate this movement into your training.

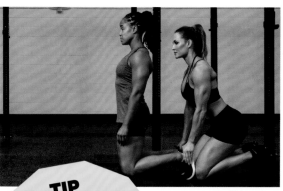

[1] Kneel down on the mat and secure your feet under a heavy piece of equipment, or have a partner hold your heels. Hold your upper body tall, with your hands positioned at your sides.

TIP

Start with low reps and work your way up to controlling your body all the way down to the floor, and pulling your body back up, using only your hamstrings.

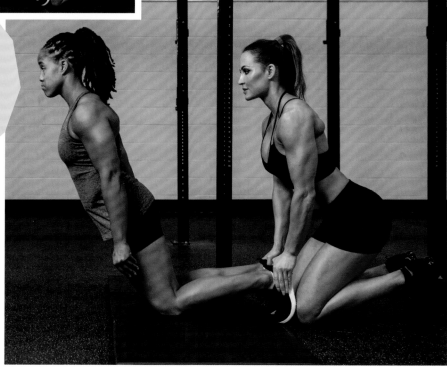

[2] Keeping your body in a straight line from your knees to your head, slowly lower your upper body down to the ground while trying to control the descent with only your hamstrings.

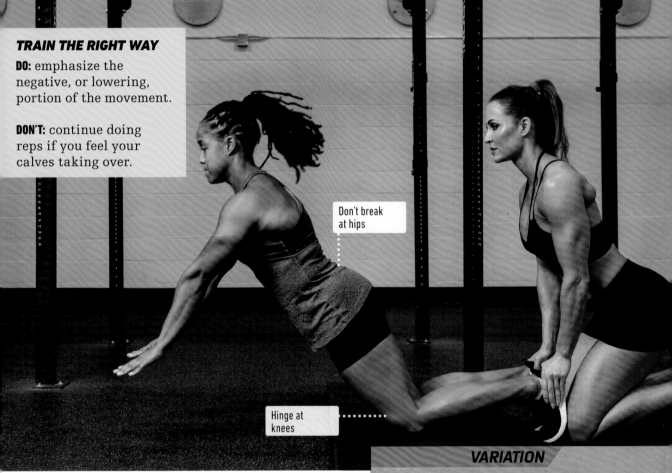

Don't break at hips

Hinge at knees

VARIATION

[3] As you get close to the floor, extend your hands out in front of you to catch yourself.

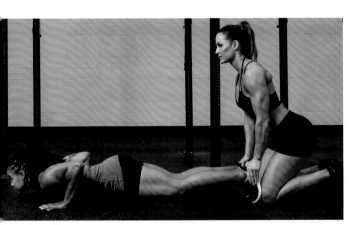

[4] Land on the ground with soft elbows. Then, from the ground, simultaneously pull with your hamstrings and forcefully push with your arms to return your body to the starting position.

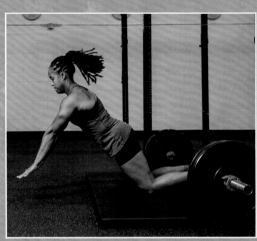

Bar-supported Nordic curl Load a bar with plates large enough that you can slide your feet under the bar. Kneel down on the mat and secure your feet under the bar, making sure the plates are anchored against the edge of the mat so they won't roll forward. Perform the movement as instructed. (This variation is great if you don't have a partner.)

SEATED LEG CURL

Compound movements can add size, but it's the isolation movements that bring out the details of a muscle, and the seated leg curl can really help sculpt the hamstring peak. To get the most out of the seated leg curl, visualize yourself pulling with the part of your hamstring you'd most like to build.

[1] Adjust the seat so your upper legs are supported by the seat and your lower legs are resting comfortably on the padded lever. Keep your legs extended, but don't lock your knees. Lower the top knee pad onto your legs.

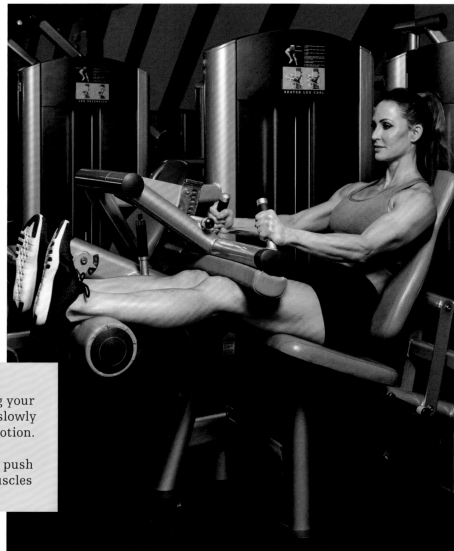

TRAIN THE RIGHT WAY

DO: focus on contracting your hamstrings and going slowly through the range of motion.

DON'T: use momentum to push the weight, as other muscles can take over.

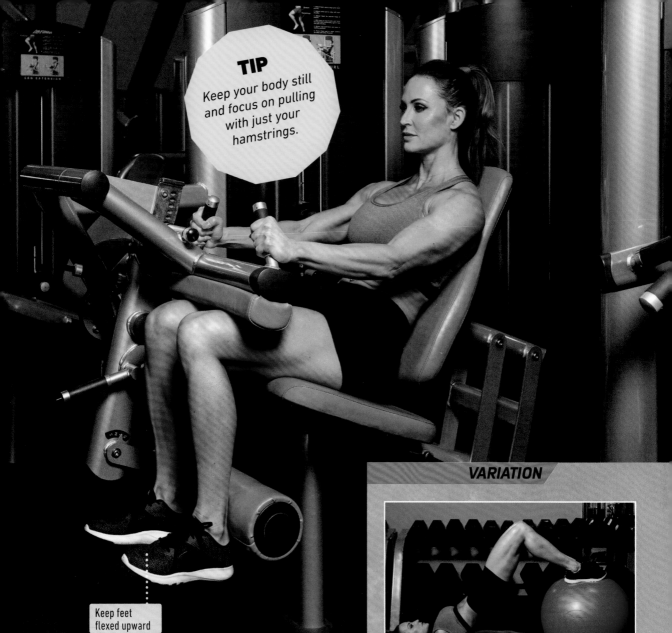

TIP
Keep your body still and focus on pulling with just your hamstrings.

Keep feet flexed upward

[2] Using equal pressure on your left and right sides, slowly squeeze your hamstrings and pull the padded lever toward you, then control the lever back to the starting position.

Stability ball hamstring curl (easier) Lie face-up on the floor and place your heels on a stability ball, with your legs extended. Place your arms at your sides with your palms facing down. Using your hamstrings, pull the stability ball toward your glutes as you extend your hips upward.

TARGETS /// calves (primary); none (secondary)
EQUIPMENT /// Smith machine with box, or standing calf raise machine

STANDING CALF RAISE

Strong calves can boost speed and strength, and the largest calf muscle in the body, the gastrocnemius, looks impressive when developed. Perform this exercise on any equipment that allows you to load the calf and get a full range of motion.

[1] Place a small box or block on the ground and under the bar. Set the bar to slightly above shoulder height. Step under the bar, placing it across your traps, and place the balls of your feet on the box. Stand up on your toes while keeping a slight bend in your knees.

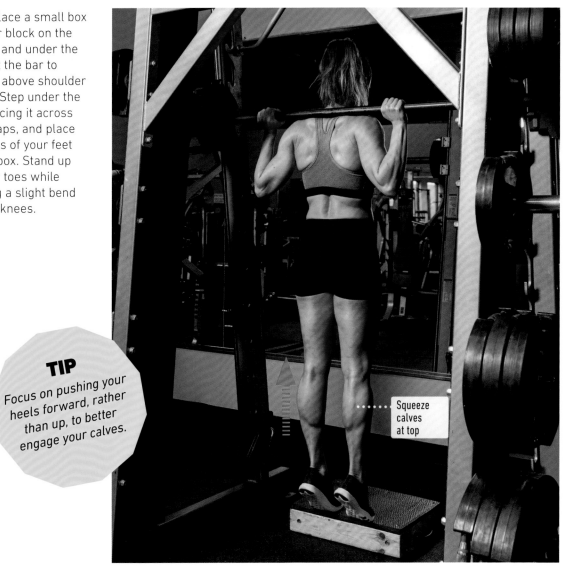

Squeeze calves at top

TIP
Focus on pushing your heels forward, rather than up, to better engage your calves.

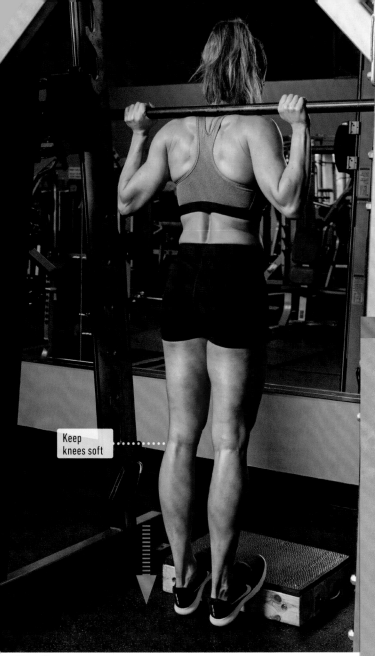

Keep knees soft

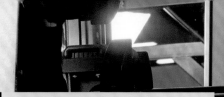

TRAIN THE RIGHT WAY

DO: keep your core tight and your upper body still throughout the rep.

DON'T: lock out your knees. (Keep your knees soft, but not bent.)

VARIATIONS

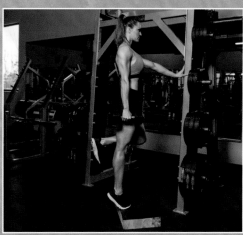

Dumbbell single-leg calf raise (easier) Stand on a box, elevating one foot behind your body. Hold a dumbbell on the same side of the working leg and grasp a sturdy object with the opposite hand. Extend your heel down and then push yourself up onto your toes. (This variation helps even out both calves.)

Leg press calf raise Place the balls of your feet on the edge of the bottom portion of the platform. Keep your legs straight and your knees soft. Unrack the safety latch and perform the exercise as you normally would. (This variation is good if you don't have access to a dedicated calf raise machine.)

[2] Engage your core, unrack the bar, and slowly lower your heels until you feel a stretch, pause momentarily, and then raise your heels until you're standing back on your toes.

SEATED CALF RAISE

Well-developed calves are the finishing touch of a balanced physique—they add curves to the legs and strength for jumps and power movements. The seated calf raise targets the soleus, a small muscle that lies under the larger gastrocnemius.

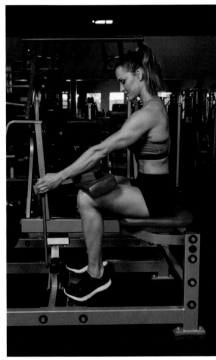

[1] Place your knees under the pads and place the balls of your feet on the platform.

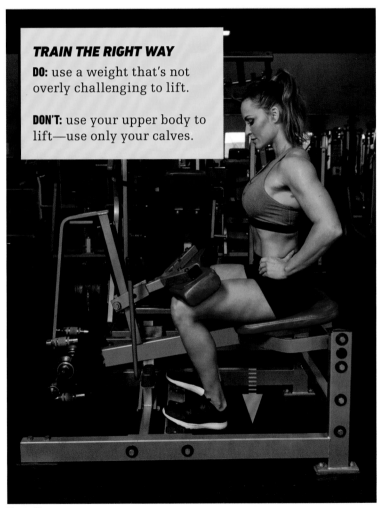

TRAIN THE RIGHT WAY

DO: use a weight that's not overly challenging to lift.

DON'T: use your upper body to lift—use only your calves.

[2] Unrack the weight and slowly allow your heels to drop into a full stretch.

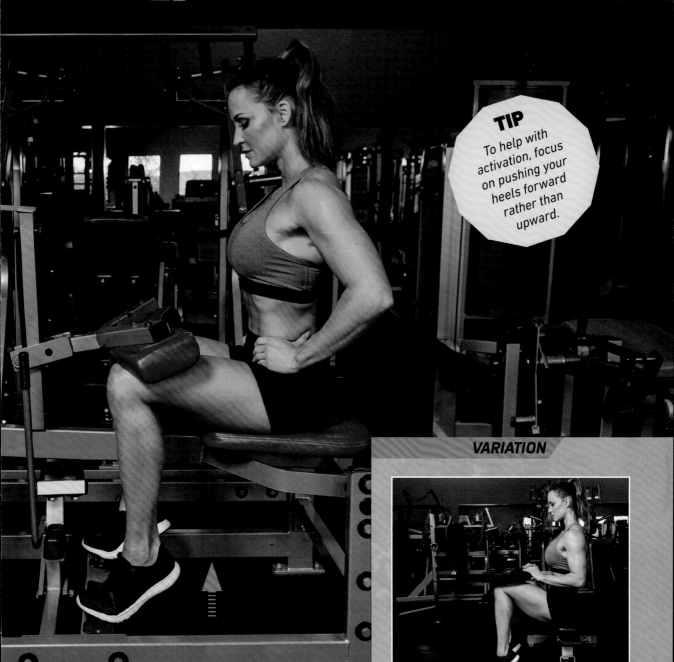

VARIATION

Seated calf raise (no machine) Place a small step or stacked plates on the ground and in front of a bench. Sit on the bench with a plate or barbell positioned across your legs and just above your knees. Place the balls of your feet on the plates or step and perform the exercise as you would on the machine.

[3] Using your calves, push the weight back up to the starting position, squeezing your calves at the top of the movement.

TARGETS **///** glutes, hamstrings, quads (primary); calves (secondary)
EQUIPMENT **///** none

LUNGE

Bodyweight exercises are a great test of stability, strength, and balance, and the lunge is no exception—it will hit almost every muscle in your legs, including the smaller stabilizer muscles. Use lunges as a warm up, as part of a workout, or add them to a circuit to help burn extra fat.

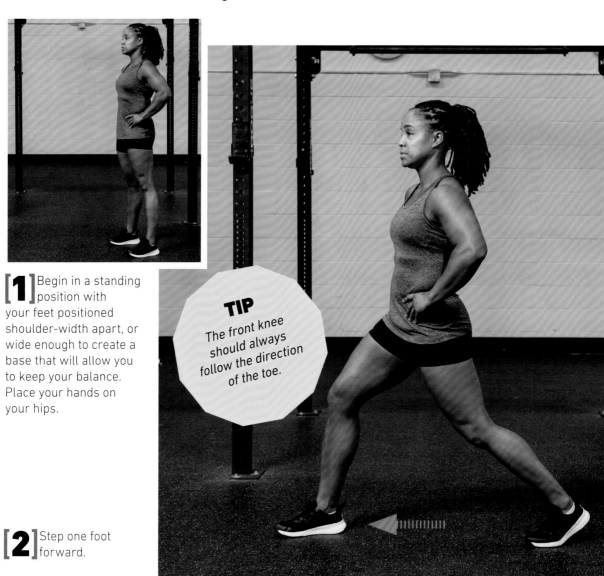

[1] Begin in a standing position with your feet positioned shoulder-width apart, or wide enough to create a base that will allow you to keep your balance. Place your hands on your hips.

TIP
The front knee should always follow the direction of the toe.

[2] Step one foot forward.

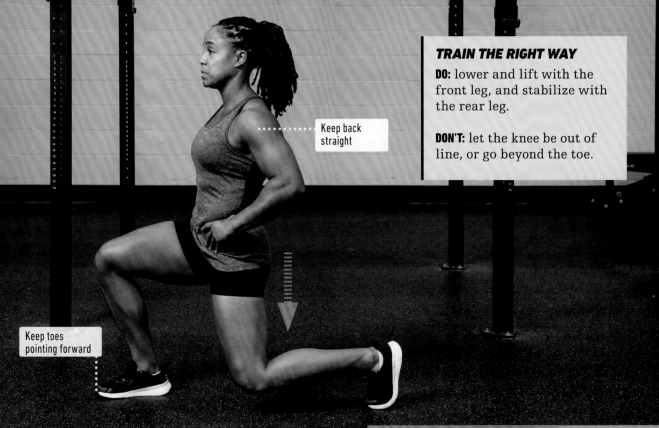

Keep back straight

Keep toes pointing forward

TRAIN THE RIGHT WAY

DO: lower and lift with the front leg, and stabilize with the rear leg.

DON'T: let the knee be out of line, or go beyond the toe.

[3] Keeping the toes of your back foot anchored to the ground, slowly lower your body down until your front upper leg reaches parallel to the ground.

[4] Push through your front heel to drive your body back up and into the starting position. Complete all reps on one side, and then repeat the movement on the opposite side.

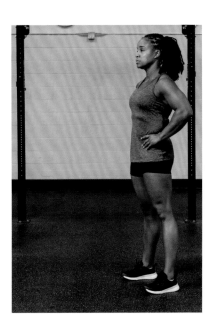

VARIATIONS

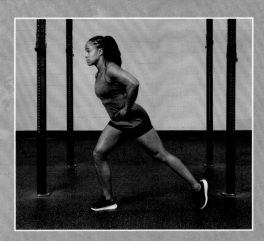

Reverse lunge Rather than taking a step forward, take one step back and lower your body down into a lunge position, performing the movement in one fluid motion. (This variation activates the glutes.)

Walking lunge Rather than remaining in one place, alternate legs and continue walking forward with each lunge.

TARGETS **///** quads (primary); none (secondary)
EQUIPMENT **///** leg extension machine

LEG EXTENSION

Perform this isolation movement to make your quad sweep pop! Quads are about 50/50 fast twitch and slow twitch muscle, so they should be trained with a combination of heavy weight with low reps, and lighter weight with higher reps.

[1] Sit on the seat of the machine and adjust the seatback so your upper legs are supported, and your lower legs fit comfortably under the lever. Brace your body by holding onto the handles.

TIP
You can target different parts of the quad by pointing your toes slightly inward or outward.

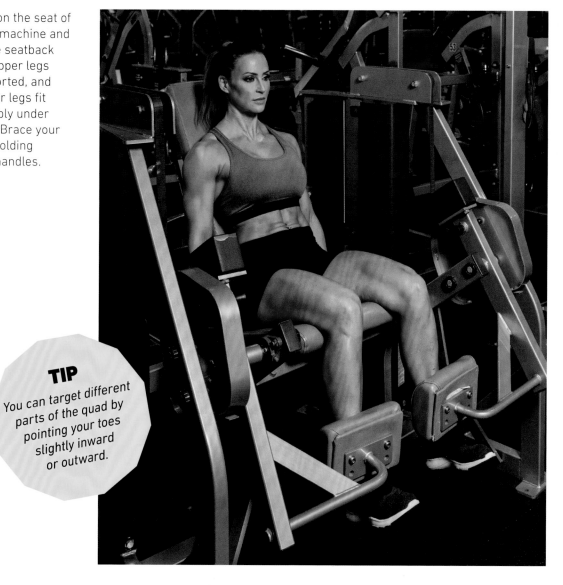

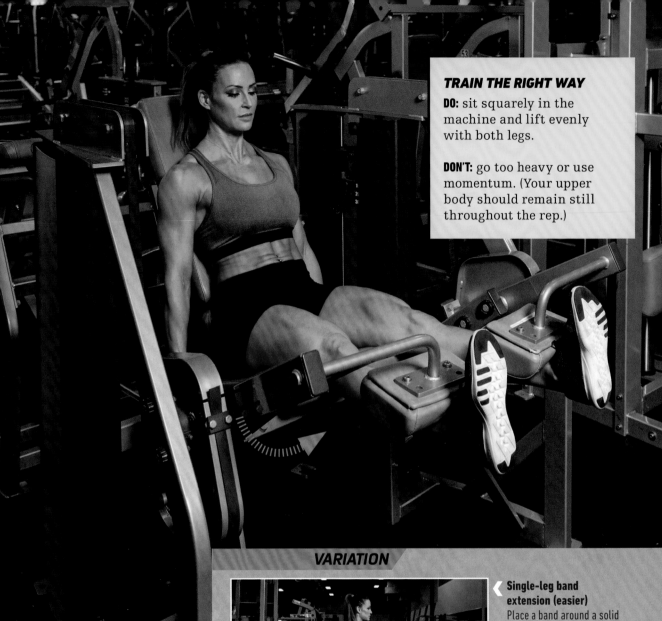

[2] Using only your quads, push the lever forward and up until your legs are fully extended, then slowly control the weight back to the starting position.

VARIATION

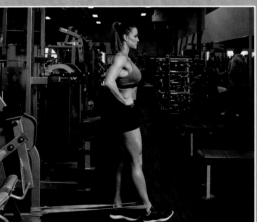

‹ Single-leg band extension (easier)
Place a band around a solid post. Loop one foot through the band and face away from the post. Extend your leg forward, just as you would with the machine leg extension.

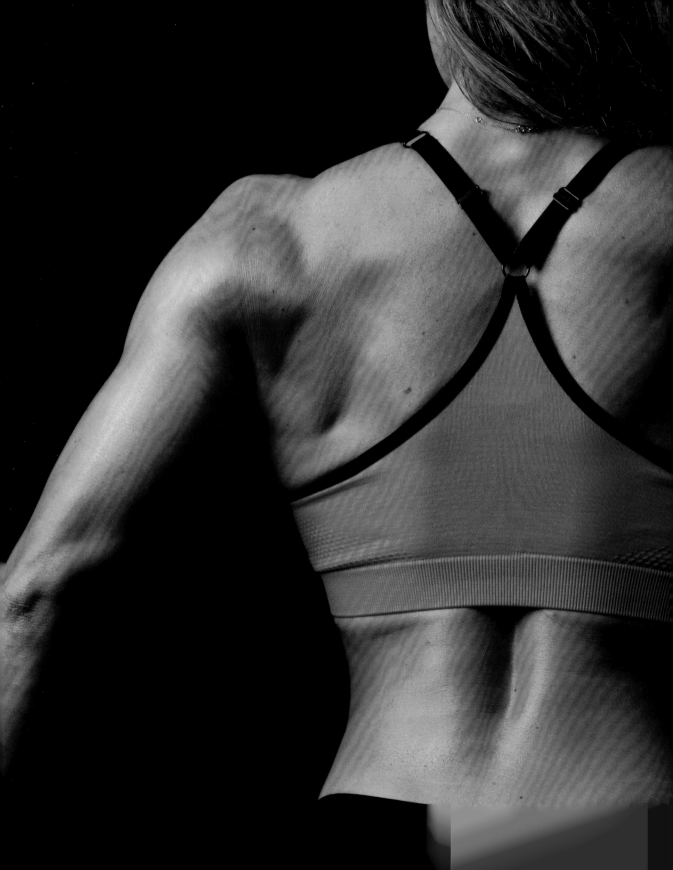

BACK

PULL-UP

The pull-up is one of the ultimate tests of strength. This total back exercise builds the lats and increases power, and as a large compound movement it can also boost metabolism. If you're not able to perform a straight pull-up, start with one of the variations and work your way up.

[1] Grasp the pull-up bar with an overhand grip and wrap your thumbs around the bar. Fully extend your arms, slightly bend your knees, and bring your feet together (or cross your legs).

TIP
Do 3 sets of as many reps as possible once or twice a week to help build strength and size.

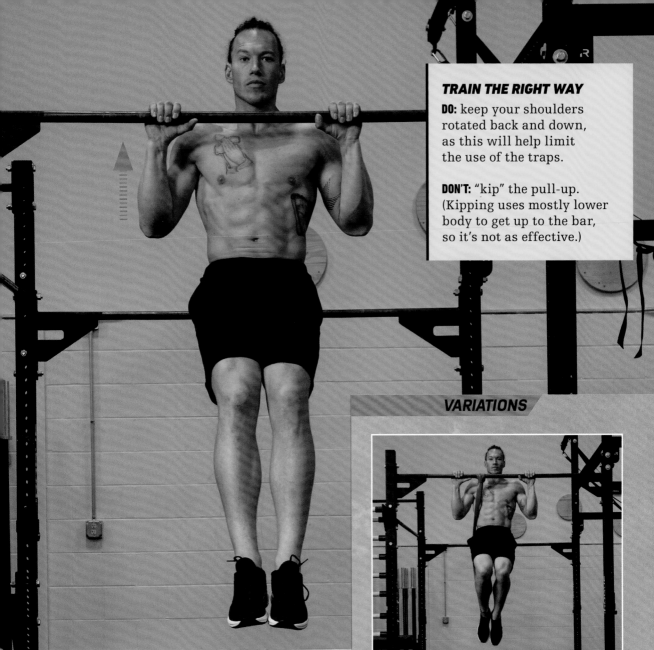

TRAIN THE RIGHT WAY

DO: keep your shoulders rotated back and down, as this will help limit the use of the traps.

DON'T: "kip" the pull-up. (Kipping uses mostly lower body to get up to the bar, so it's not as effective.)

VARIATIONS

[2] From a dead hang, engage your lats and pull yourself up until your chin reaches the bar, pause, and then slowly lower yourself back down to the starting position.

Band-assisted pull-up (easier) Secure a resistance band to the pull-up bar and place one foot in the loop to assist with the pull-up.

Machine-assisted pull-up with alternating negatives (easier) Set your desired weight on an assisted pull-up machine and place your knees on the platform. Perform a pull-up with both hands, then alternate with single arm negatives. (This will help build strength and help you progress to a full pull-up.)

TARGETS /// lats, rhomboids, traps (primary); biceps, abs(secondary)
EQUIPMENT /// cable machine and v-bar attachment

CLOSE-GRIP LAT PULLDOWN

A staple in any bodybuilder's training regimen is the lat pulldown, which helps shape a v-taper by building your upper lats to make your waist appear smaller, and your physique appear more symmetrical. Pulldowns can make pull-ups easier and increase overall strength for deadlifts and squats.

[1] Sit on the bench with your feet flat on the ground. Grasp the v-bar handle and secure your knees under the knee pad. Rotate your shoulders back and down, keeping your wrists straight and your elbows in.

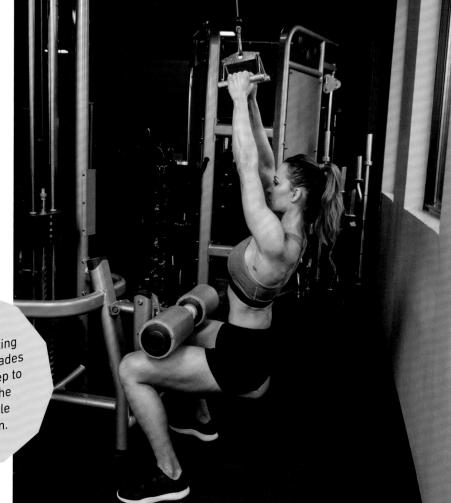

TIP
Focus on squeezing your shoulder blades together mid-rep to strengthen the mind-muscle connection.

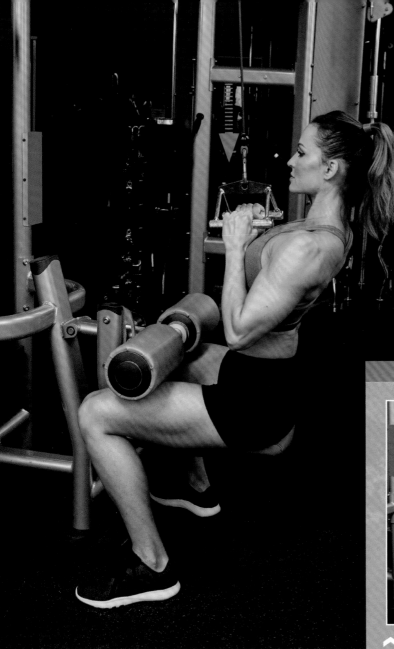

TRAIN THE RIGHT WAY

DO: pause at the eccentric (negative) point of the exercise to keep tension in the muscle.

DON'T: use momentum to move the weight, which will work the shoulders and lower back.

VARIATIONS

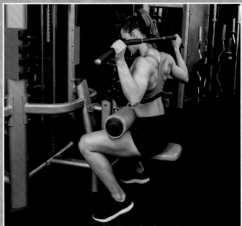

Behind-the-neck pulldown Use the wide straight bar attachment and 50% of your normal weight lifted. Lean forward and rotate your shoulders back. Grasp the bar with an overhand grip and pull the bar behind your head to mid-neck height. Use only the lower two-thirds range of motion and do not fully extend the bar. (This is great for developing upper mid-back depth.)

Wide-grip lat pulldown Use the wide straight bar handle and an overhand grip. Pull the bar to just above your collarbone. (This better engages the outer lats.)

[2] Lean back slightly as you pull the handle toward your chest, pause briefly when the handle is just above your chest, then slowly release the weight back to the starting position.

TARGETS **///** lats, rhomboids, traps (primary); biceps, abs (secondary)
EQUIPMENT **///** high-pulley cable with handle attachment

SINGLE-ARM PULLDOWN

Every bodybuilder has muscle imbalances, but unilateral (single-arm or single-leg) exercises like the single-arm pulldown can help even out asymmetries and create a more aesthetic physique, help prevent injury, and improve strength.

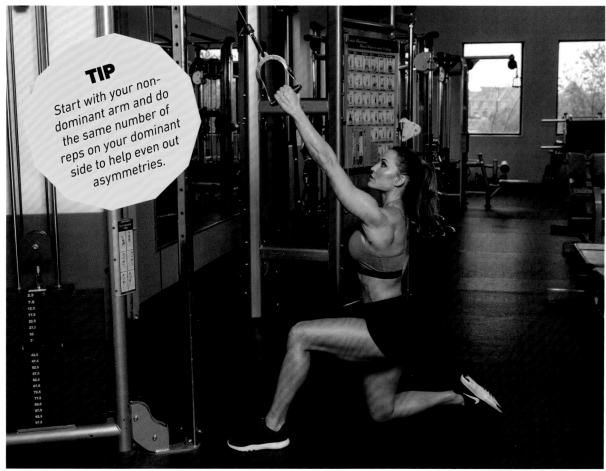

TIP
Start with your non-dominant arm and do the same number of reps on your dominant side to help even out asymmetries.

[1] Grasp the handle and drop into a lunge position with your lead leg mirroring the arm that's working, and the knee of your trail leg placed on the floor. Rotate your shoulders back and down, keep your wrist straight, and your elbow pulled in. Place your nonworking hand on your hip.

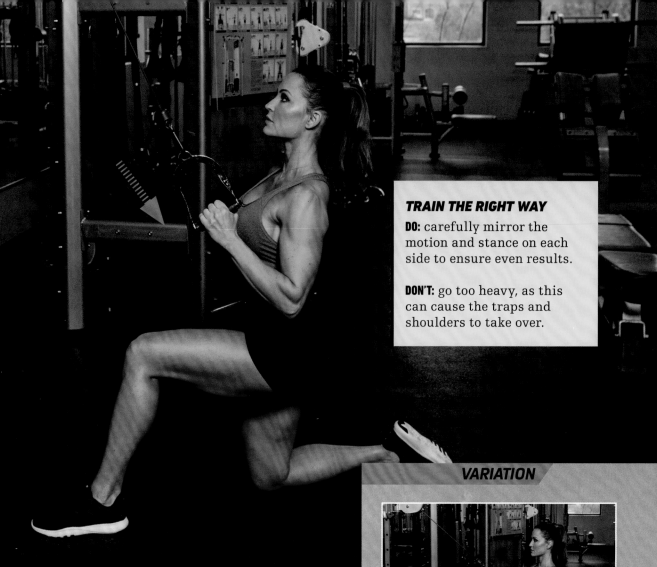

[2] Pull the handle down until your hand reaches your chest, pause, and then control the handle back to the starting position.

VARIATION

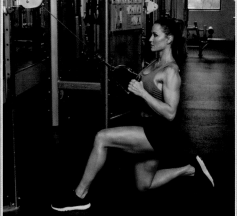

Single-arm pulldown from chest height Adjust the cable to standing chest height, drop into a lunge, and perform the exercise as instructed. (This angle targets more of the mid-back.)

TARGETS /// middle lats, rhomboids, traps (primary); biceps, forearms (secondary)
EQUIPMENT /// Olympic bar and plates

BENT-OVER BARBELL ROW

One of the six basic lifts, this movement adds definition and width to the middle back, and can be performed in a variety of ways. Master this one and you'll strengthen your other lifts, improve posture, and make your waist look smaller.

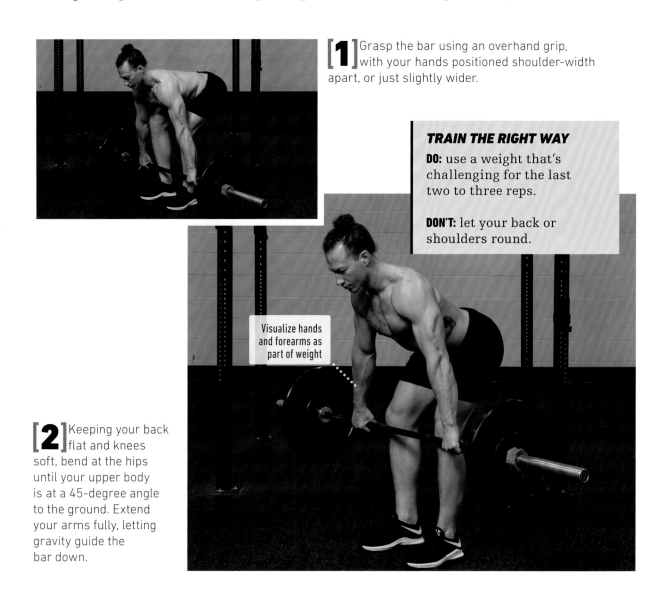

[1] Grasp the bar using an overhand grip, with your hands positioned shoulder-width apart, or just slightly wider.

TRAIN THE RIGHT WAY

DO: use a weight that's challenging for the last two to three reps.

DON'T: let your back or shoulders round.

Visualize hands and forearms as part of weight

[2] Keeping your back flat and knees soft, bend at the hips until your upper body is at a 45-degree angle to the ground. Extend your arms fully, letting gravity guide the bar down.

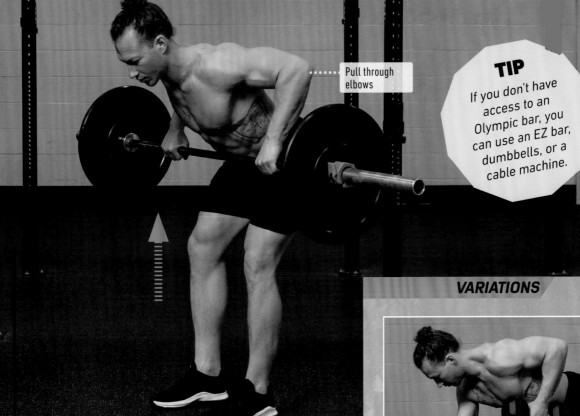

Pull through elbows

TIP

If you don't have access to an Olympic bar, you can use an EZ bar, dumbbells, or a cable machine.

[3] With your shoulders square and elbows pulled in, pull the bar toward your chest. Pause just before the bar touches your chest.

[4] Lower the bar back down to the starting position in a controlled fashion.

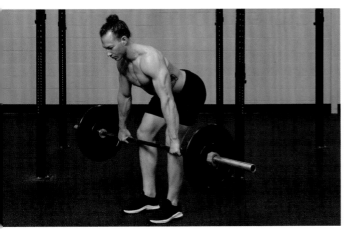

VARIATIONS

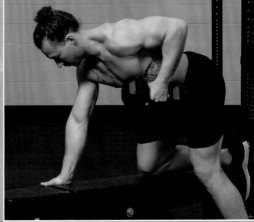

▲ **Single-arm bent-over row** Hold a dumbbell with a neutral grip and place your opposite knee on a flat bench. Your other leg should remain straight and the foot should be flat on the ground. Lean forward and place your free hand firmly on the bench. With a tight core and flat back, pull the dumbbell to your ribcage, keeping your elbows in. (This variation is good for minimizing muscle imbalances.)

Underhand grip row Hold the bar with an underhand grip. (The form and range of motion are the same, but this grip better targets the biceps.)

Chest-supported row Adjust the bench to a 45-degree incline and lie face-down on the bench. Have a spotter hand you the bar and, using an overhand or underhand grip, perform the row with your elbows pulled in and your chest pressed against the bench the entire time. (This variation targets more of the upper back.)

TARGETS **///** lats, outer lats, lower traps (primary); lower back, rear delts, biceps (secondary)
EQUIPMENT **///** barbell, small plates, v-bar attachment

T-BAR ROW

This staple of classic-era bodybuilding will develop width and definition, and hit every muscle in the back. You can experiment with angles and grips to specialize this exercise—standing taller will target the upper lats, while bending the upper body to a 45-degree angle will target the lower lats.

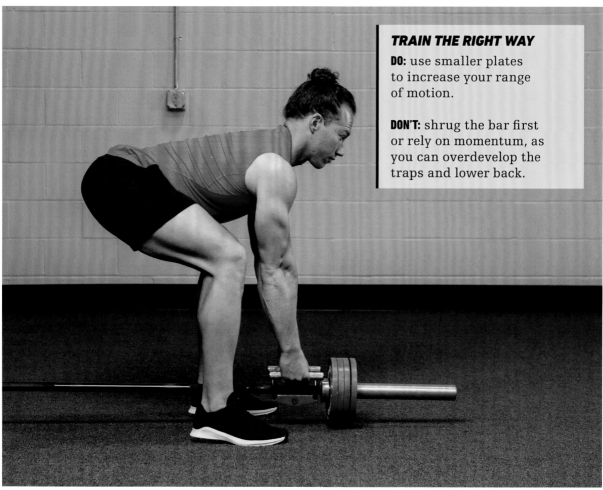

TRAIN THE RIGHT WAY

DO: use smaller plates to increase your range of motion.

DON'T: shrug the bar first or rely on momentum, as you can overdevelop the traps and lower back.

[1] Secure an Olympic bar in a sturdy corner or t-bar station, and load the weights onto the end of the bar. Facing away from the bar, straddle the bar with your feet positioned shoulder-width apart, and place a v-bar attachment underneath and near the far end of the bar, with the Olympic bar positioned in the center of the "v". Grasp the v-bar handle with a neutral grip.

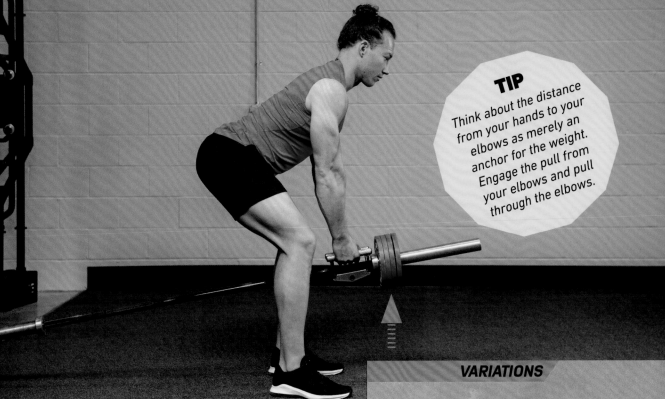

TIP

Think about the distance from your hands to your elbows as merely an anchor for the weight. Engage the pull from your elbows and pull through the elbows.

[2] Keeping your back flat, use only your legs to pull the bar up off the ground while keeping your arms fully extended, your knees bent, hips hinged, and your upper body positioned at a 45-degree angle.

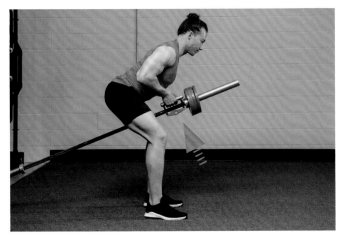

[3] Keeping your elbows pulled in, slowly pull the bar toward your chest until the plates nearly touch your chest, and then slowly control the weight back down until your arms are once again fully extended.

VARIATIONS

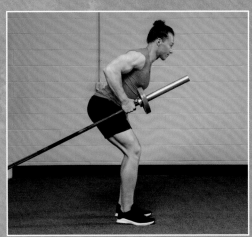

Single-arm t-bar row (easier) Using about 40% of the weight you'd normally use, stand to one side of the bar and use a neutral grip to grasp the bar. Pull the bar to your chest. After the set is complete on one side, step over the bar and repeat on the opposite side.

Chest-supported t-bar row Step onto a t-bar row machine and rest your chest against the pad, grab the handles, and unrack the bar. Pull through your full range of motion like you would with the traditional t-bar row. (This variation can be used when a traditional t-bar row station isn't available.)

TARGETS /// lats, rhomboids, traps (primary); lower back, biceps (secondary)
EQUIPMENT /// adjustable bench and dumbbells

SUPINE DUMBBELL ROW

The upper middle back can be difficult to target, but this exercise does the job well. The bench provides support and limits the use of momentum, which can shift focus to unintended muscle groups, and using dumbbells ensures you'll get an even pull on both sides to help build a symmetrical back.

[1] Adjust the bench to a 45-degree angle. Hold the dumbbells with a neutral grip, and lie stomach-down on the bench with your feet firmly planted on the floor.

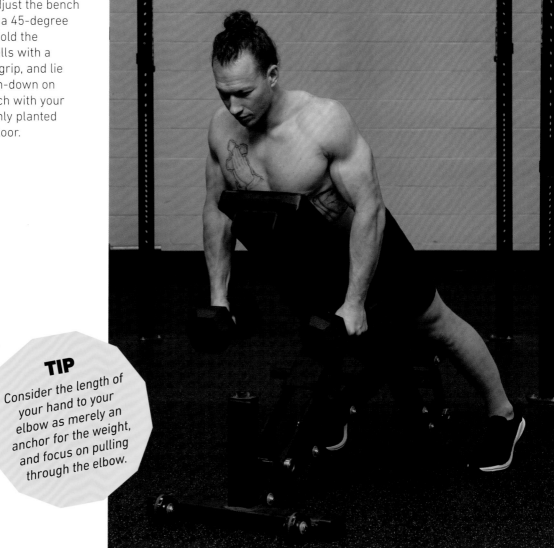

TIP
Consider the length of your hand to your elbow as merely an anchor for the weight, and focus on pulling through the elbow.

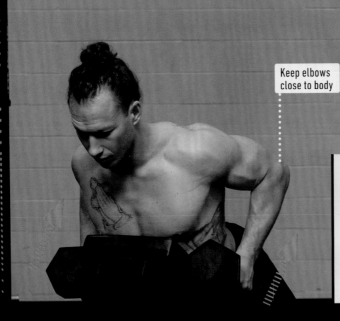

Keep elbows close to body

TRAIN THE RIGHT WAY

DO: keep your chest pressed against the bench throughout the entire movement.

DON'T: shrug the weights first, as this will recruit mostly the traps to do the lifting.

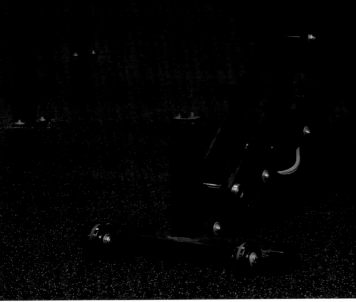

[2] Pull the dumbbells upward and slightly back, squeezing your back at the top of the rep, and then slowly lower the dumbbells back down to the starting point.

VARIATION

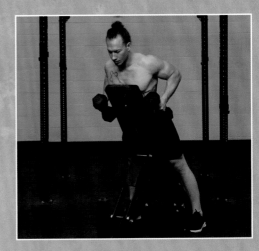

High incline supine row Adjust the bench to a 60-degree angle and perform the exercise as instructed (This variation targets the upper lats, rhomboids, and rear delts.)

TARGETS /// rhomboids, traps, lats (primary); biceps (secondary)
EQUIPMENT /// cable row station and double-D handle attachment

CABLE ROW

An aesthetic back requires attention to developing width and depth—the lats contribute width, but the rhomboids and traps fill out the back to create a rippling masterpiece of strength and proportion. The cable row can help add this dimension by applying constant tension to the muscles.

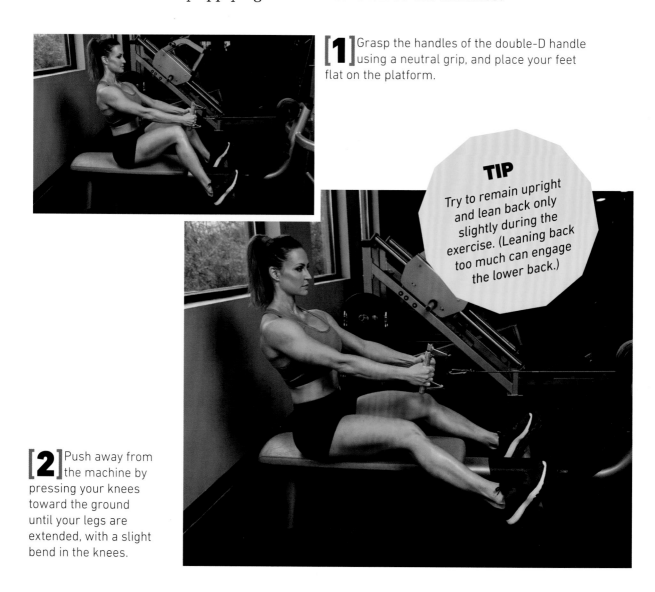

[1] Grasp the handles of the double-D handle using a neutral grip, and place your feet flat on the platform.

TIP

Try to remain upright and lean back only slightly during the exercise. (Leaning back too much can engage the lower back.)

[2] Push away from the machine by pressing your knees toward the ground until your legs are extended, with a slight bend in the knees.

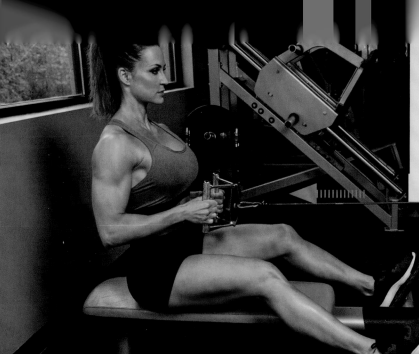

TRAIN THE RIGHT WAY

DO: pull through the elbow, keep your wrists straight, and keep your forearms parallel to the ground.

DON'T: lean back more than 15 degrees to perpindicular.

[3] Sit tall and engage your core. Extend your shoulders forward slightly and pull the handle back until it reaches your chest, rotating your shoulders back as you pull through a comfortable, full range of motion.

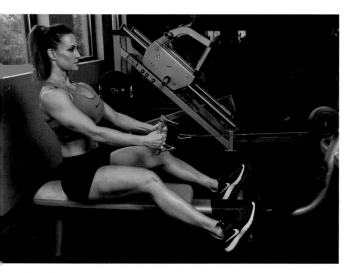

[4] Use your back to slowly control the weight back to the starting position, pausing mid-rep and squeezing your shoulder blades together before returning the weight all the way back to the starting position.

VARIATIONS

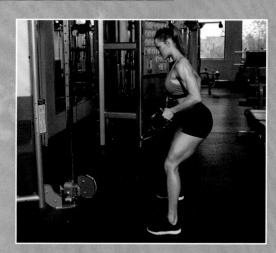

Single-arm cable row Adjust a single cable to the lowest pin and use the handle attachment. Grasp the handle with a neutral grip and stand with feet slightly wider than shoulder-width. Pull the handle to your midsection. (This variation works the lower lats).

Low-pulley cable row If you don't have access to a cable row station, place a 45lb plate in front of a single cable placed on the lowest pin and attach the v-bar handle. Grasp the handle, brace your heels against the plate, and lower yourself down to the ground. Perform the row as you would on the cable row station. (This variation targets the lower lats and back.)

TARGETS /// upper lats, mid lats, traps, lower back (primary); glutes, hamstrings, abs (secondary)
EQUIPMENT /// barbell, plates, squat rack or power rack

RACK PULL

Also known as a partial deadlift, the rack pull is the second stage of a deadlift where the effort switches from pushing with the legs to pulling with the mid- and upper back. Not only will this exercise improve your overall strength, it will add depth and width to your back.

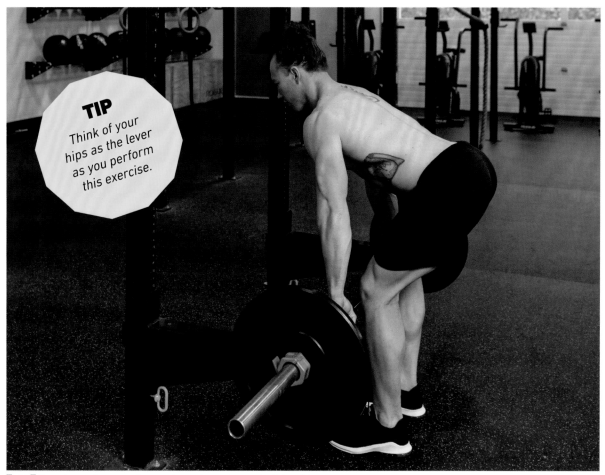

TIP
Think of your hips as the lever as you perform this exercise.

[1] Set the safety on the rack to about knee-height. (If you are taller, you can go slightly above the knee.) Place the barbell on the rack and place the plates on the bar. Grasp the bar using an overhand grip that is 50 percent wider than shoulder-width, keeping your shoulders square, your knees slightly bent, and your arms extended. Unrack the bar.

Keep shoulders high ··········

Keep back and core tight

Keep hips low

VARIATIONS

Dumbbell partial pull (easier) Start with an overhand grip with the dumbbells in front of your body. Bend your hips and lean forward until your upper body reaches a 45-degree angle and the dumbbells are at knee-height. Keeping your arms extended, pull the dumbbells up while pushing your hips forward.

Speed pull (more challenging) Set up the rack like you would for traditional rack pulls. On the "pull" portion, power up the weight and focus on being explosive, and then slowly lower the weight back down. (This is a good variation for building speed and power.)

[2] Pull the bar upward while simultaneously extending your hips forward until your legs are fully extended, pause momentarily, then slowly lower the bar back down to the starting position.

DUMBBELL PULLOVER

This is one of Arnold Schwarzenegger's favorite exercises and one of the only movements that trains antagonist (or opposing) muscle groups. It targets the outer lats, upper chest, and gives a good stretch while doing so. If you're looking to build an epic physique, this exercise should be on your must-do list!

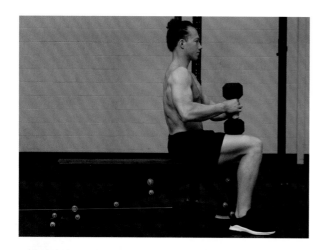

TRAIN THE RIGHT WAY

DO: keep your hips down and tuck your chin slightly.

DON'T: go too heavy on these, as it's easy for your form to break down.

[1] Sit on the end of the bench and place the dumbbell on your thigh. Wrap your thumbs around the handle and brace your palms against the end of the dumbbell.

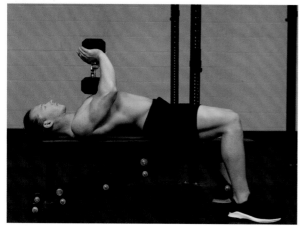

[2] "Kick" the dumbbell back to your chest as you lie back on the bench, keeping your glutes and back pressed flat against the bench, and your feet flat on the floor. Tuck your chin slightly to your chest.

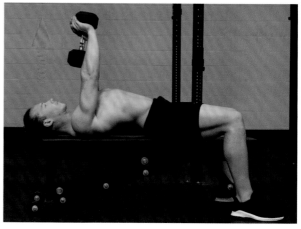

[3] Keeping your elbows in, extend your arms to push the dumbbell directly over your chest.

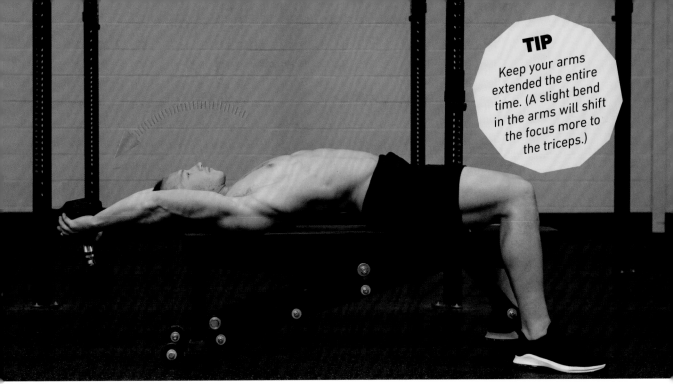

TIP
Keep your arms extended the entire time. (A slight bend in the arms will shift the focus more to the triceps.)

[4] Slowly extend the dumbbell back and downward until you feel a stretch in your lats.

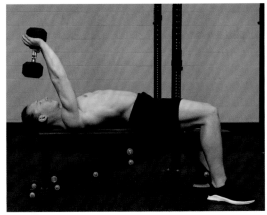

[5] Pull the dumbbell back to just before the starting point. (You should still feel a stretch in your lats.)

VARIATIONS

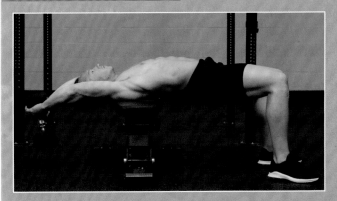

Cross-bench pullover Lie across the bench with your shoulders pinned to the bench, and your feet flat on the floor. Arch your back slightly and perform the exercise as instructed. (This variation can give you a better stretch, and is better for taller athletes.)

Single-arm pullover (easier) Hold a light dumbbell in one hand and extend your arm backwards until you feel a stretch. Complete all reps on one side and then switch to the opposite arm.

Straight-arm pushdown (easier) Attach a straight bar to a high-pulley cable. Grasp the bar using an overhand grip with your hands slightly wider than shoulder-width apart. Lean forward at a 30-degree angle, engage your lats, and push the bar down to your knees.

TARGETS /// lats, traps, rhomboids (primary); biceps, forearms, abs (secondary)
EQUIPMENT /// squat rack or power rack, Olympic bar

INVERTED ROW

This highly customizable exercise improves systemic strength, helps prevent injury, and can be done almost anywhere. Key benefits include enhancing the strength and overall musculature of the back, increasing grip strength, and improving core stability.

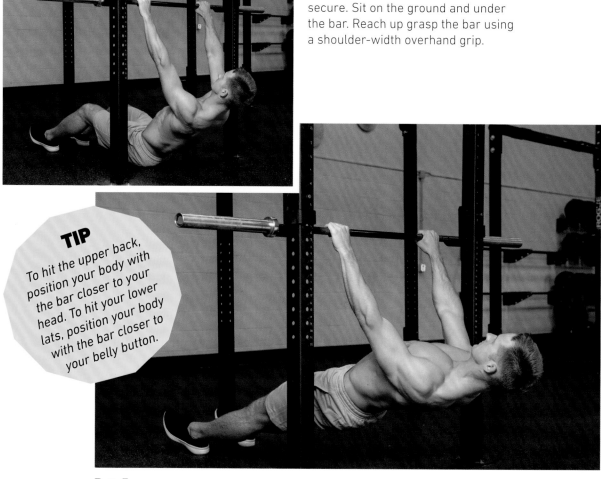

[1] Place the bar about hip height on the rack and make sure it's secure. Sit on the ground and under the bar. Reach up grasp the bar using a shoulder-width overhand grip.

TIP
To hit the upper back, position your body with the bar closer to your head. To hit your lower lats, position your body with the bar closer to your belly button.

[2] Extend your feet out in front of you and pull your body up and into a plank position, with your legs extended straight out and your weight resting in your heels.

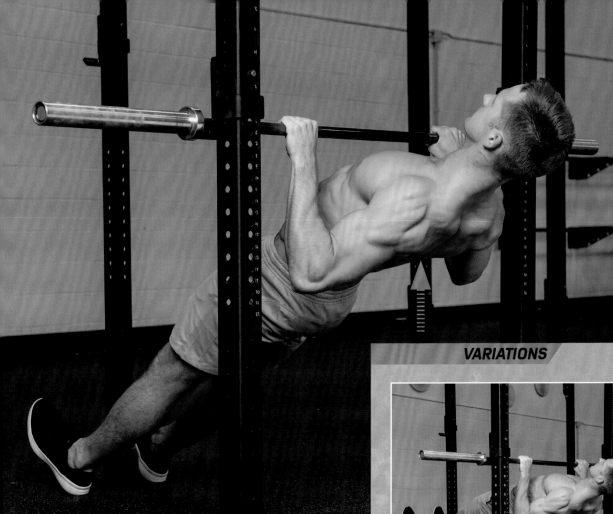

TRAIN THE RIGHT WAY

DO: keep your body in the plank position for the entire exercise.

DON'T: allow your hips to drop or your shoulders to shrug while pulling yourself up.

Feet-elevated inverted row (more challenging)
Place a bench in front of you and about 4 inches (10cm) away from your feet. Get into the row position and set your feet on top of the bench. Perform the exercise as instructed.

Wide-grip inverted row (more challenging) Place your hands twice as wide as normal. (This will help target the outer part of the lats.)

Underhand-grip inverted row Wrap your hands under the bar, instead of over the bar. (This variation targets the biceps, especially when you wrap your thumbs around the bar.)

[3] Focusing on your back, slowly pull your body up until your chest touches the bar, keeping your forearms straight, your elbows close to your body, your shoulders flat and square, and your body in a plank position. Lower your body back down until your arms are fully extended.

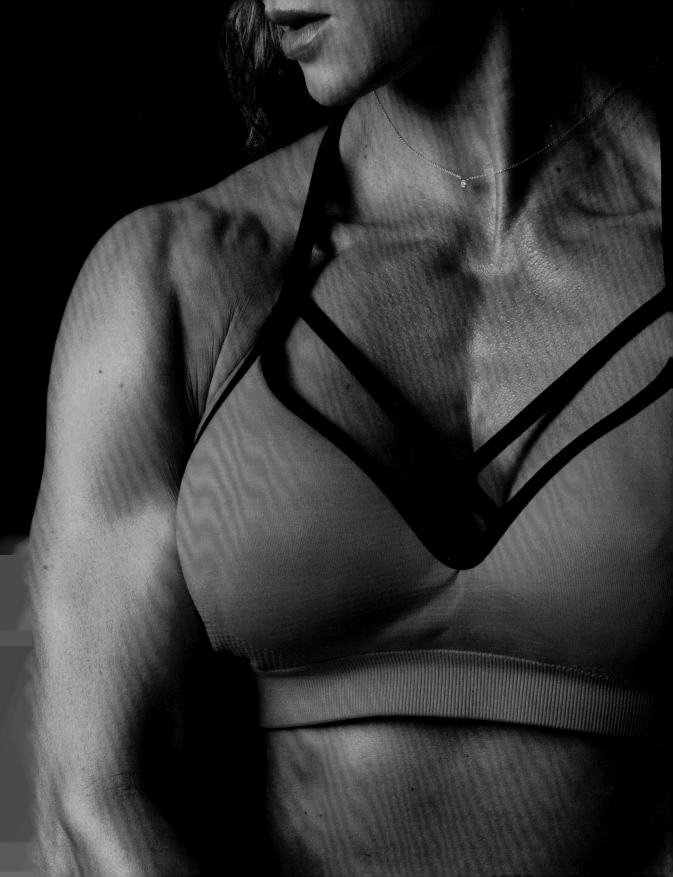

CHEST

TARGETS /// pectorals, front delts, triceps (primary); lats, abs (secondary)
EQUIPMENT /// bench, barbell, and plates

BENCH PRESS

Master this exercise and you'll gain upper body power and strength. A well-developed chest ties the shoulders to the rest of the physique, and lends to the appearance of a smaller waist.

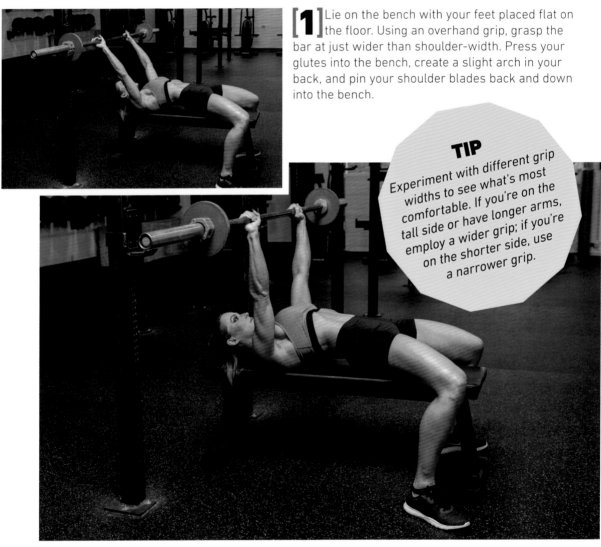

[1] Lie on the bench with your feet placed flat on the floor. Using an overhand grip, grasp the bar at just wider than shoulder-width. Press your glutes into the bench, create a slight arch in your back, and pin your shoulder blades back and down into the bench.

TIP

Experiment with different grip widths to see what's most comfortable. If you're on the tall side or have longer arms, employ a wider grip; if you're on the shorter side, use a narrower grip.

[2] Keeping your core tight, engage your lats to pull the bar from rack.

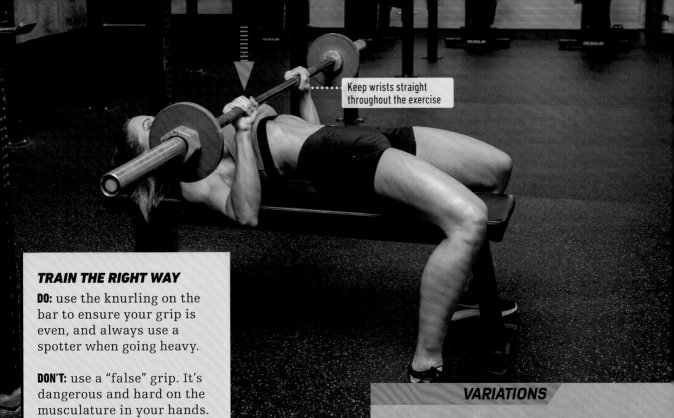

Keep wrists straight throughout the exercise

TRAIN THE RIGHT WAY

DO: use the knurling on the bar to ensure your grip is even, and always use a spotter when going heavy.

DON'T: use a "false" grip. It's dangerous and hard on the musculature in your hands.

[3] Slowly "pull" the bar toward your chest, making sure to keep your shoulder blades pinned to the bench and your elbows pulled in tightly. Lower the bar to a point just before it touches your chest, then pause momentarily.

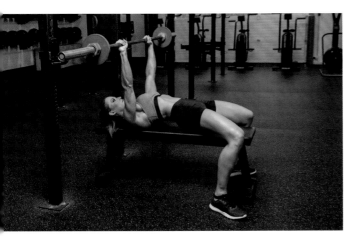

[4] Press the bar back up until your arms are fully extended. (The motion of the rep should follow a slight arc.)

VARIATIONS

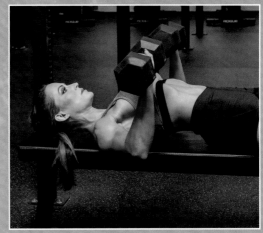

Dumbbell bench press Use dumbbells and follow the same guidelines for form and range of motion. (Dumbbells allow you to train both sides evenly, and can help increase your strength for the barbell bench press. This variation also is good if you don't have a spotter to assist the lift.)

Single-arm dumbbell press Choose a dumbbell that's 20% lighter than you'd normally use. Start with your nondominant side, place your feet wider than normal, and counterbalance the movement with your opposite arm. (This variation can improve core strength and help with muscle imbalances.)

TARGETS **///** upper chest (primary); middle chest, triceps (secondary)
EQUIPMENT **///** adjustable bench and dumbbells

DUMBBELL INCLINE BENCH PRESS

A well-developed upper chest is an integral part of a balanced upper body. Strong, full shoulders are complemented by, and flow well with, a full upper chest. During leaning, muscle is often lost from the upper body, which can leave a gaunt-looking physique, but this movement can counteract that.

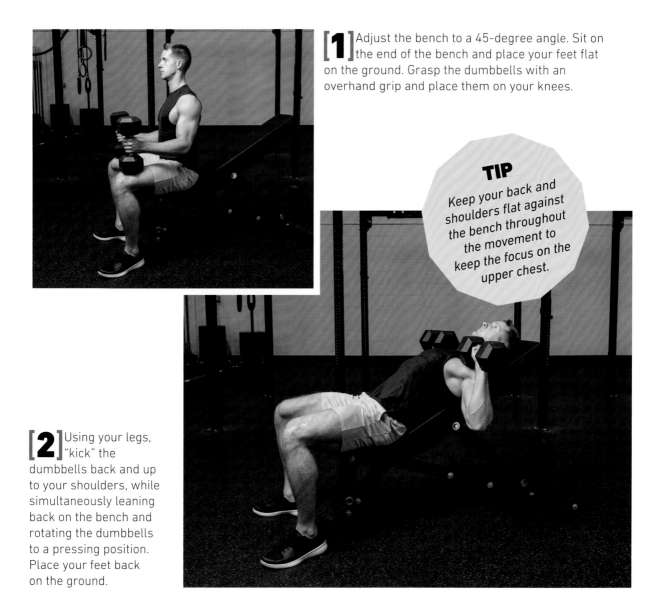

[1] Adjust the bench to a 45-degree angle. Sit on the end of the bench and place your feet flat on the ground. Grasp the dumbbells with an overhand grip and place them on your knees.

TIP

Keep your back and shoulders flat against the bench throughout the movement to keep the focus on the upper chest.

[2] Using your legs, "kick" the dumbbells back and up to your shoulders, while simultaneously leaning back on the bench and rotating the dumbbells to a pressing position. Place your feet back on the ground.

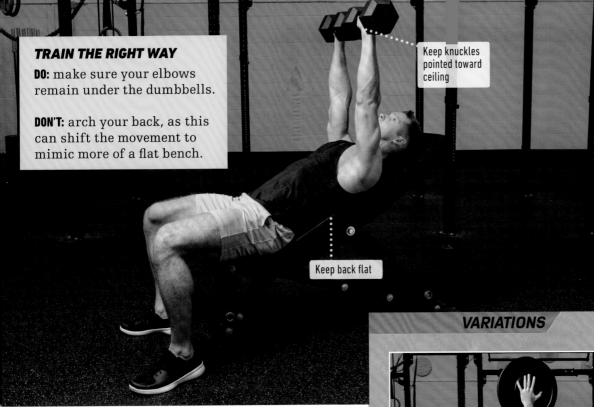

TRAIN THE RIGHT WAY

DO: make sure your elbows remain under the dumbbells.

DON'T: arch your back, as this can shift the movement to mimic more of a flat bench.

Keep knuckles pointed toward ceiling

Keep back flat

[3] Press the dumbbells upward while rotating them slightly inward.

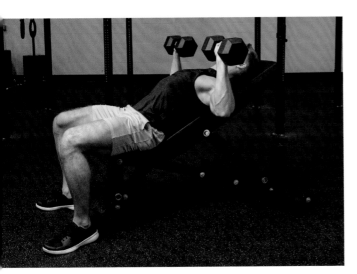

[4] Slowly lower them back down until your upper arms are just below parallel to the ground.

VARIATIONS

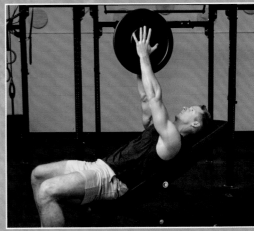

Incline plate press Hold a plate upright, so your hands are close together. Keeping your elbows as close together as possible, press the plate upward while squeezing your chest. (This variation targets the middle upper chest.)

Barbell incline bench press Use collars to secure the plates to the bar. Use your lats to unrack the bar, lower the bar to just above your chest, and then press the bar back up and slightly back until your arms are fully extended.

High incline bench press (more challenging) Adjust the bench to a 60- or 70-degree angle, and use a slightly lighter weight than you'd use for a traditional incline bench. (This variation is especially effective for building muscle just under the collarbone, and for building the front delts.)

TARGETS /// chest, anterior delts (primary); triceps (secondary)
EQUIPMENT /// cable pulley and handle attachment

CROSS-BODY CHEST PRESS

Few exercises can create definition and strong curves in the chest like the cross-body chest press. You have the ability to focus on one side at a time and also control the contraction mid-rep, and the result is a seamless integration with the delts and an improved overall physique balance.

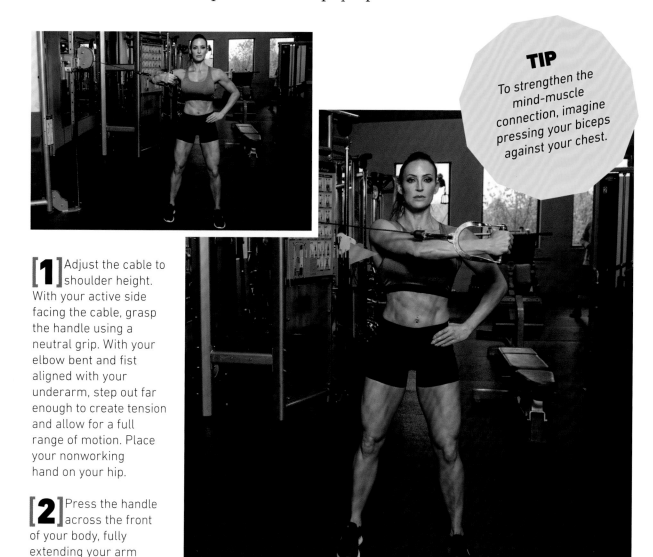

TIP

To strengthen the mind-muscle connection, imagine pressing your biceps against your chest.

[1] Adjust the cable to shoulder height. With your active side facing the cable, grasp the handle using a neutral grip. With your elbow bent and fist aligned with your underarm, step out far enough to create tension and allow for a full range of motion. Place your nonworking hand on your hip.

[2] Press the handle across the front of your body, fully extending your arm at the top of the movement.

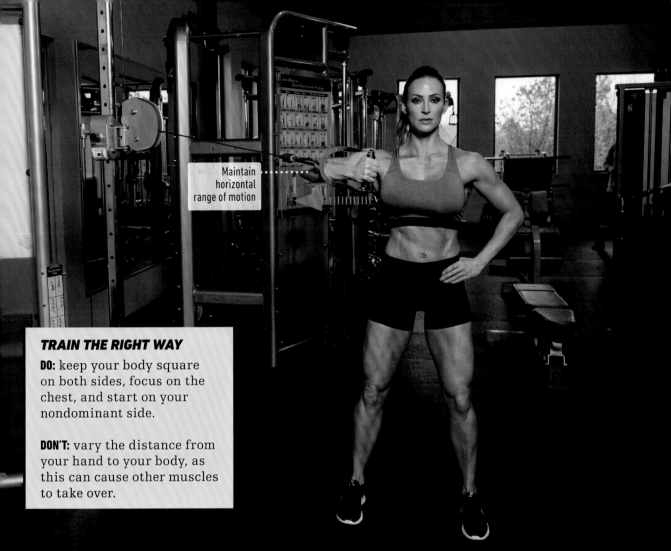

Maintain horizontal range of motion

TRAIN THE RIGHT WAY

DO: keep your body square on both sides, focus on the chest, and start on your nondominant side.

DON'T: vary the distance from your hand to your body, as this can cause other muscles to take over.

[3] Slowly control the handle back to the starting position. Complete a full set on one side, then switch to the opposite side.

VARIATION

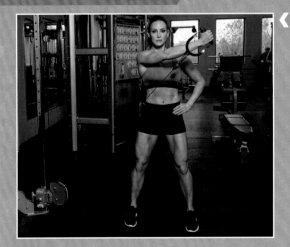

❮ **Low-to-high cross-body press** Adjust the cable to the lowest position. Start with a bend in your elbow and a neutral grip. Press the handle up and across your body. (This variation targets more of the lower chest and shoulders.)

TARGETS /// upper chest, anterior delts (primary); triceps, core (secondary)
EQUIPMENT /// bench or plyo box

DECLINE PUSH-UP

By changing the angle of the traditional push-up, the decline push-up effectively targets the upper chest to help develop muscle in an area that tends to look hollow when leaning down. A well-developed upper chest ties the shoulders into the rest of the upper body, as well.

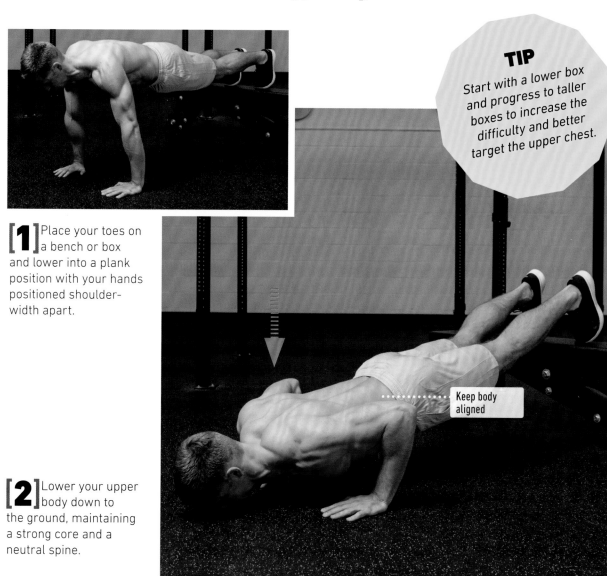

TIP
Start with a lower box and progress to taller boxes to increase the difficulty and better target the upper chest.

[1] Place your toes on a bench or box and lower into a plank position with your hands positioned shoulder-width apart.

Keep body aligned

[2] Lower your upper body down to the ground, maintaining a strong core and a neutral spine.

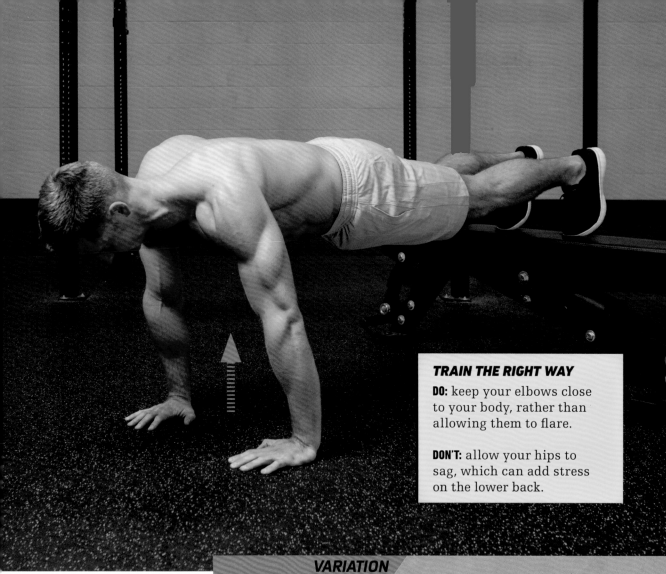

[3] Using your chest and shoulders, press yourself back up to the starting position.

VARIATION

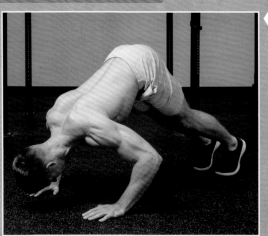

Pike push-up (easier)
Drop into a pike position with your arms extended. Rise up onto your toes, keeping your legs straight. Perform the push-up as you normally would. (This variation is perfect for beginners or to use as a finisher.)

TARGETS /// upper chest (primary); triceps, forearms (secondary)
EQUIPMENT /// cable machine and handle attachments

INCLINE CABLE FLYE

Only a few exercises can build and tone the upper chest, but the incline cable flye is at the top of the list. A full upper chest ties the shoulders in to the rest of the physique and can help improve strength and power.

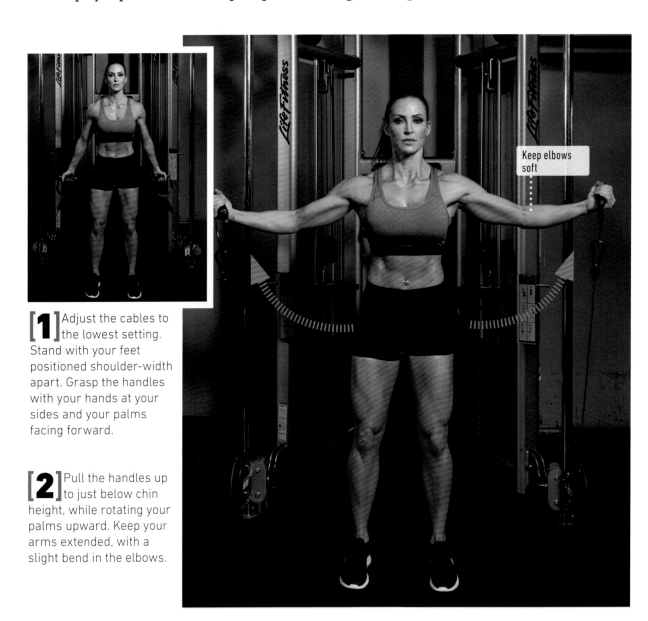

Keep elbows soft

[1] Adjust the cables to the lowest setting. Stand with your feet positioned shoulder-width apart. Grasp the handles with your hands at your sides and your palms facing forward.

[2] Pull the handles up to just below chin height, while rotating your palms upward. Keep your arms extended, with a slight bend in the elbows.

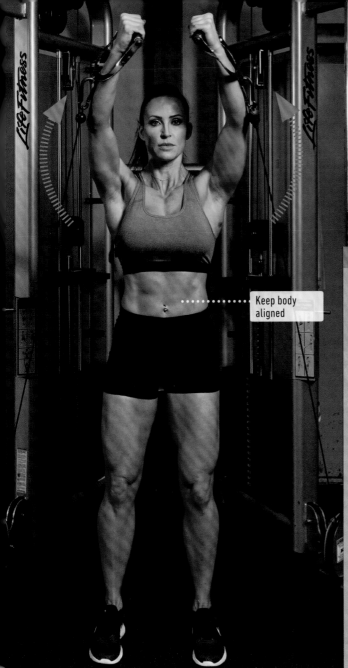

Keep body
aligned

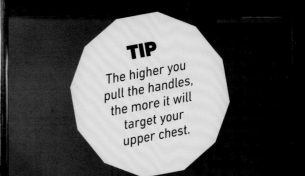

TIP
The higher you pull the handles, the more it will target your upper chest.

VARIATIONS

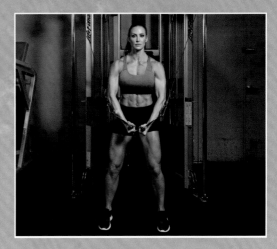

Decline cable flye Adjust the cables to the highest setting and pull the handles to just below chin height. Pull the cables down in an arcing motion until your hands nearly touch, pause, then slowly return the cables to the position just below chin height. (Keep a slight bend in the elbows at all times.)

Incline bench flye (easier) Adjust the bench to a 60-degree angle. Sit squarely on the bench with your feet flat on the ground. Hold the dumbbells using a neutral grip, lay back, and extend the dumbbells straight up. Slowly lower the dumbbells out to your sides, then return them to the starting position.

Flat bench flye (easier) Hold dumbbells using a neutral grip and lie back on a flat bench. Extend the dumbbells upward and directly over your mid-chest. Slowly extend your arms outward and toward the ground, pause, and then push the dumbbells back to the starting position. Keep a slight bend in your elbows throughout the exercise. (Think about hugging a barrel.)

[3] Keeping a tight core, pull the cables out and up in an arcing motion until your hands are above your head, pause momentarily, then slowly return the cables to the starting position.

TARGETS **///** chest (primary); triceps, front delts (secondary)
EQUIPMENT **///** dip bar or dip chair

DIPS

Dips train the chest, shoulders, and triceps, and can help the upper body musculature flow better aesthetically and also improve strength for upper body pressing exercises. You can customize this exercise to suit your skill level and match your training goals by slightly changing angles.

[1] Grasp the handles of a dip chair or dip bar using a neutral grip. Jump up so your arms are extended and your body is balanced over your arms. Lean forward slightly and bend your legs at your knees. (If needed, extend your legs backward to counterbalance your upper body.)

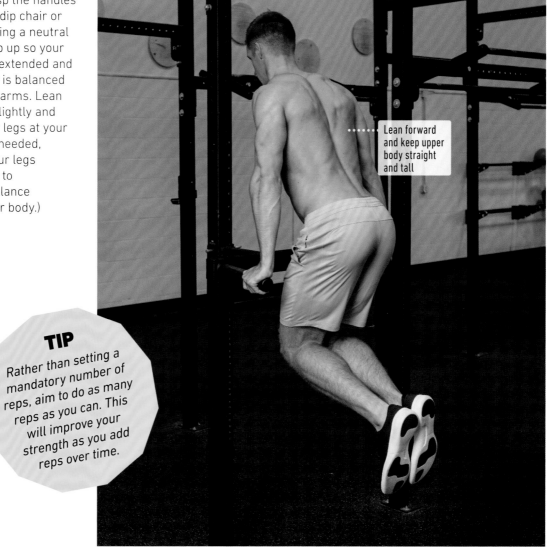

Lean forward and keep upper body straight and tall

TIP
Rather than setting a mandatory number of reps, aim to do as many reps as you can. This will improve your strength as you add reps over time.

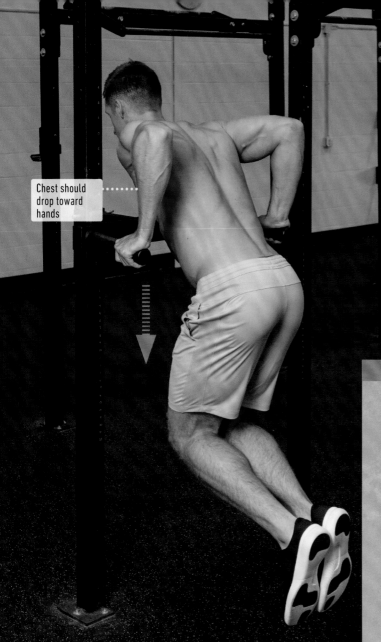

Chest should drop toward hands

[2] Rotate your shoulders back and down, and slowly lower your body down until you feel a stretch in your chest and shoulders. Pause at the bottom of the movement, then push your body back up to the starting position.

VARIATIONS

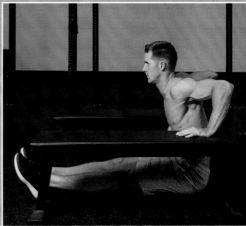

Between-benches dips (easier) Place two benches parallel to each other and about 2 to 3 feet (.6m to .9m) apart. Stand between the benches and place one hand on each bench. With legs and arms extended, toes pointed, heels on the ground, and elbows pulled in slightly, lower your body down between the benches.

Machine-assisted dips (easier) Set the weight on a dip machine to an amount that challenges you, but allows you to perform at least six reps. Place your knees on the knee pad and perform the exercise as you would for bodyweight dips. (This is a good variation for beginners.)

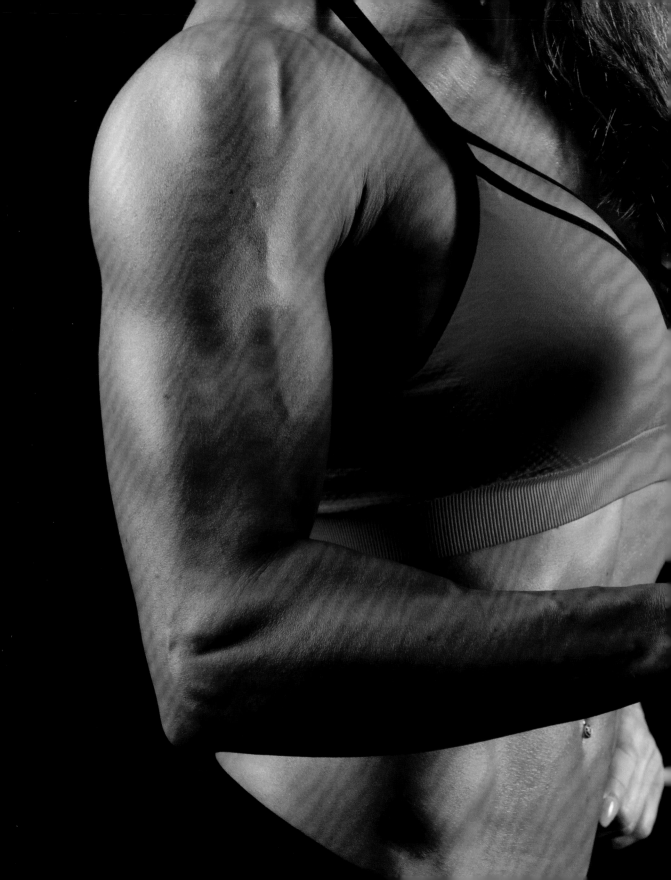

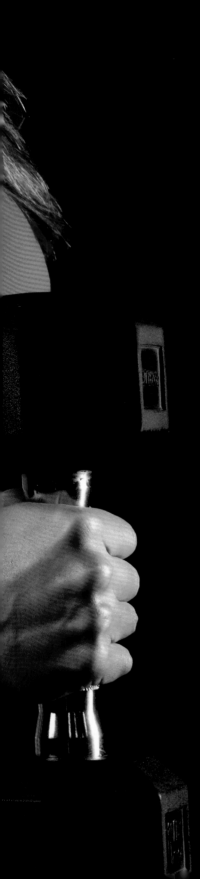

ARMS

TARGETS **///** triceps (primary); chest, shoulders (secondary)
EQUIPMENT **///** bench, barbell, and plates

CLOSE-GRIP BENCH PRESS

A variation of the traditional bench press, the close-grip bench press will help improve your pressing power for other lifts, and will develop both strength and definition. Opt for a lighter weight to maintain proper form, and keep the focus on lifting the weight with just your triceps.

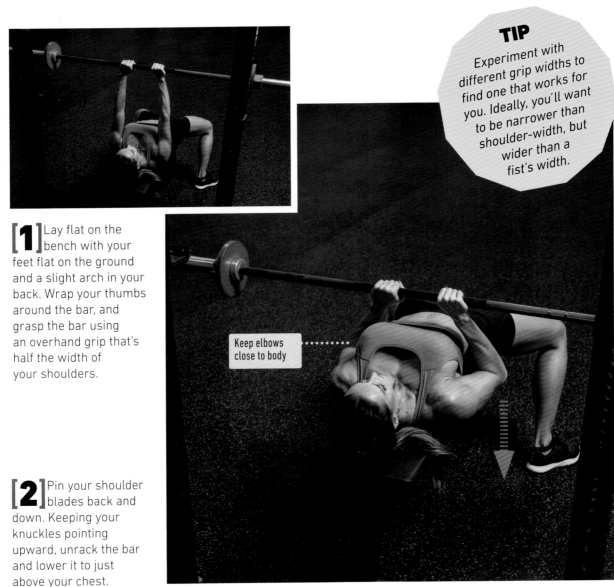

TIP
Experiment with different grip widths to find one that works for you. Ideally, you'll want to be narrower than shoulder-width, but wider than a fist's width.

[1] Lay flat on the bench with your feet flat on the ground and a slight arch in your back. Wrap your thumbs around the bar, and grasp the bar using an overhand grip that's half the width of your shoulders.

Keep elbows close to body

[2] Pin your shoulder blades back and down. Keeping your knuckles pointing upward, unrack the bar and lower it to just above your chest.

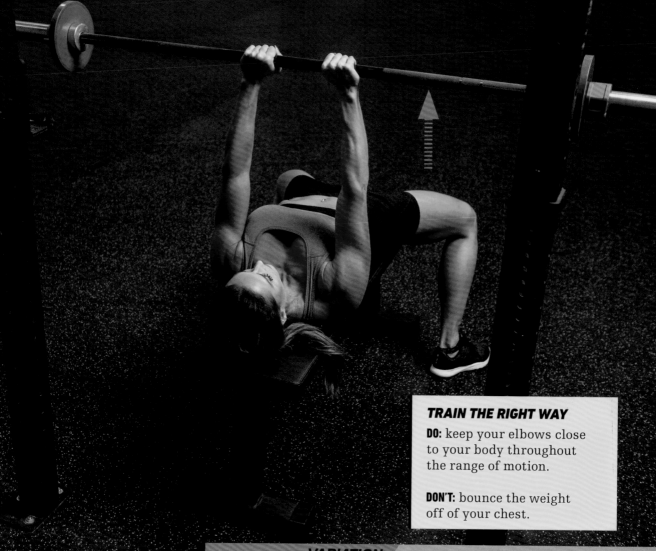

TRAIN THE RIGHT WAY

DO: keep your elbows close to your body throughout the range of motion.

DON'T: bounce the weight off of your chest.

[**3**] Press the bar upward and slightly back until your arms are fully extended. Pause momentarily, then return the bar to the starting position.

VARIATION

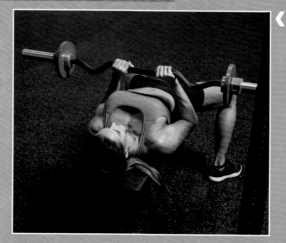

Close-grip EZ bar press Lie flat on a bench as you hoist the bar over your chest. Use a narrow grip and perform the exercise as instructed. (This variation is great as a burn out or finisher, and may help lifters who have existing wrist issues.)

TARGETS /// triceps (primary); chest, shoulders (secondary)
EQUIPMENT /// bench

BENCH DIPS

Bench dips will sculpt your triceps, and can help tie the physique together aesthetically, as your shoulders and chest work in unison with your triceps. These can be scaled to be very easy or very difficult, depending on your strength level and if you're using them as a starting exercise or a finisher.

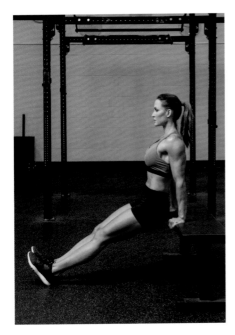

[1] Place your palms on the edge of the bench with your fingers facing forward and your arms fully extended. Extend your legs out in front of you, with your weight resting in your heels. (Your body should be positioned about one inch (2.5cm) from the edge of the bench.)

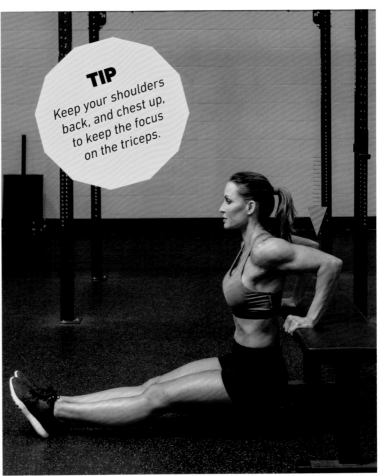

TIP
Keep your shoulders back, and chest up, to keep the focus on the triceps.

[2] Slowly lower your body down until you feel a stretch in your chest. Keep your upper body tall, and your elbows pointing backward and positioned close to your body.

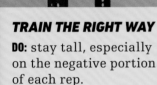
[3] Engage your triceps to push your body back up into the starting position.

VARIATIONS

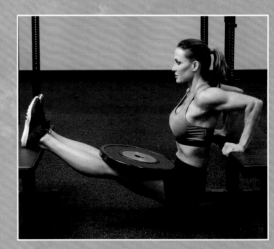

Weighted feet-elevated bench dips (more challenging) Position two benches about one leg's-length distance apart. Secure your hands on the first bench, place your heels on the second bench with your legs fully extended, and place a plate on your lap and above your knees. (The range of motion is the same as standard bench dips.)

Feet-elevated bench dips (more challenging) Secure your hands on the first bench, place your heels on the second bench with your legs fully extended, and perform the exercise as you would for standard bench dips.

TARGETS /// biceps (primary); forearms (secondary)
EQUIPMENT /// dumbbells

STANDING BICEPS CURL

A well-chiseled arm has strong curves, from shoulder to forearm, and this time-tested classic does the trick. Strong biceps can help with overall strength, especially when it comes to pull-downs and chin-ups.

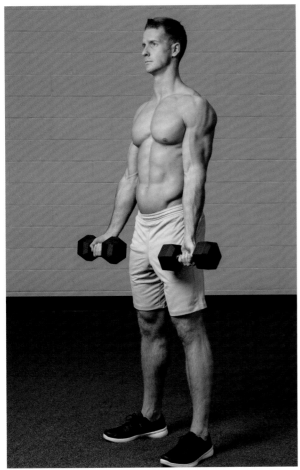

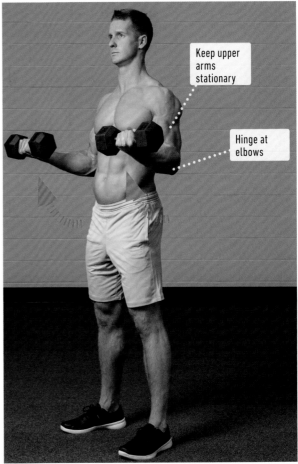

Keep upper arms stationary

Hinge at elbows

[1] Stand with soft knees and your feet positioned shoulder-width apart. Hold the dumbbells slightly out in front of you, using an underhand grip.

[2] Keeping your shoulders back and your wrists straight, pull the dumbbells up toward your chest by contracting the biceps and flexing at the elbows. Pause slightly just before your forearms are perpendicular to the ground.

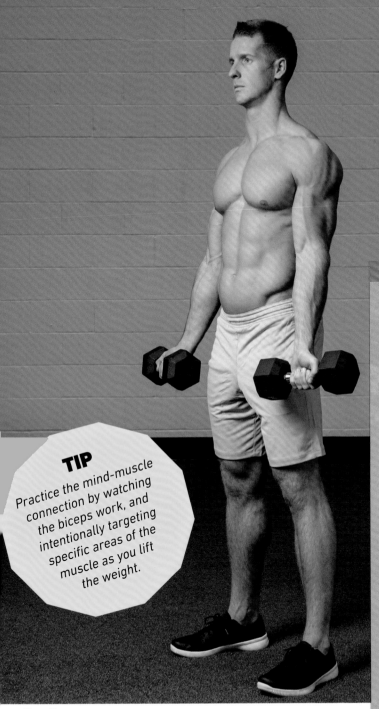

VARIATIONS

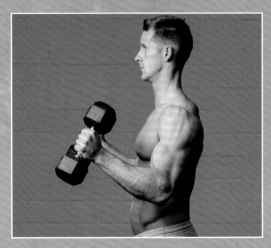

Hammer curl Hold the dumbbells with a neutral grip, and curl as you would normally. (This can be done either seated or standing.)

Seated dumbbell curl (more challenging) Sit on a bench with your feet together and flat on the ground. Keep your upper arms stationary, use an underhand grip, and hold your arms slightly away from your body to allow for a full range of motion.

EZ bar partial-rep curl Sit on a bench with your feet flat on the ground and positioned slightly in front of you. Grasp the EZ bar with an underhand grip and hold it just above your knees. Curl the bar, stopping just before the forearm reaches perpendicular at the top, and just before the bar touches your knees at the bottom.

TIP

Practice the mind-muscle connection by watching the biceps work, and intentionally targeting specific areas of the muscle as you lift the weight.

[3] Slowly lower the weight back down to the starting position.

TARGETS **///** biceps (primary); forearms (secondary)
EQUIPMENT **///** EZ bar and plates

EZ BAR DRAG CURL

This classic move targets the biceps with a range of motion that is different from other curls. It effectively isolates the biceps from the shoulders and helps sculpt and grow the biceps more quickly than can be done with traditional curls.

[1] Hold an EZ bar with a shoulder-width, underhand grip. Extend your arms downward and position the bar in front of your thighs.

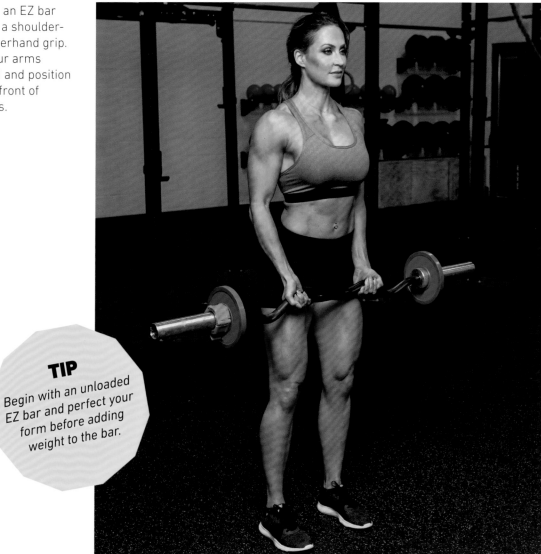

TIP
Begin with an unloaded EZ bar and perfect your form before adding weight to the bar.

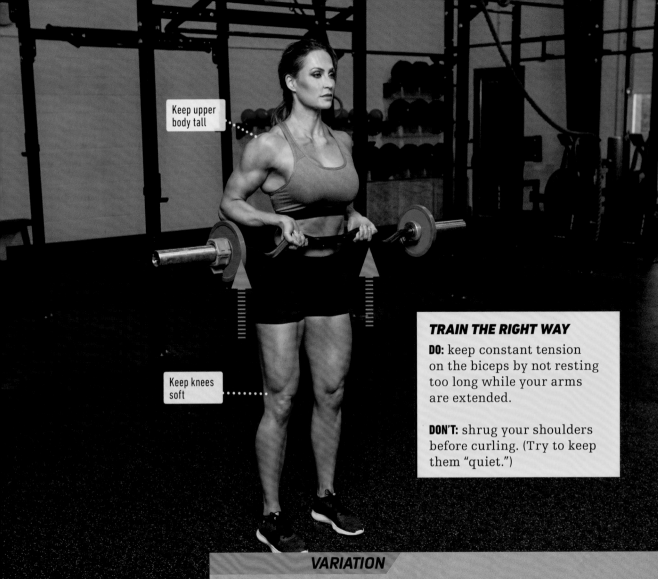

Keep upper
body tall

Keep knees
soft

TRAIN THE RIGHT WAY

DO: keep constant tension on the biceps by not resting too long while your arms are extended.

DON'T: shrug your shoulders before curling. (Try to keep them "quiet.")

[2] Slowly bend your elbows and pull, or "drag," the bar upwards and along the front of your body, pause when the bar reaches your upper midsection, then slowly lower the bar back down to the starting position.

VARIATION

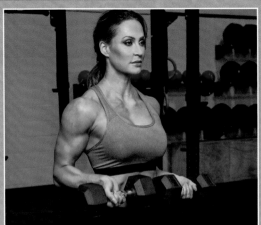

❮ **Dumbbell drag curl** Hold the dumbbells against your thighs using an underhand grip, keeping a bend in the wrists. Perform the exercise as you would with the EZ bar, making sure to keep the dumbbells even on both sides. (This variation is good for eliminating muscle imbalances.)

SPIDER CURL

If you have strong shoulders it can be difficult to isolate the biceps. Take those stronger muscle groups out of the mix and create beautiful biceps peaks with this unique exercise that really isolates the biceps.

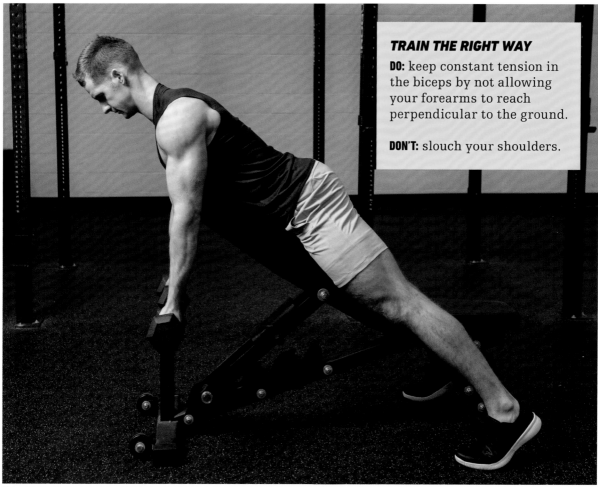

TRAIN THE RIGHT WAY

DO: keep constant tension in the biceps by not allowing your forearms to reach perpendicular to the ground.

DON'T: slouch your shoulders.

[1] Adjust the bench to a 45-degree angle and lie stomach-down on the bench. Hold the dumbbells using an underhand grip and extend your arms toward the ground.

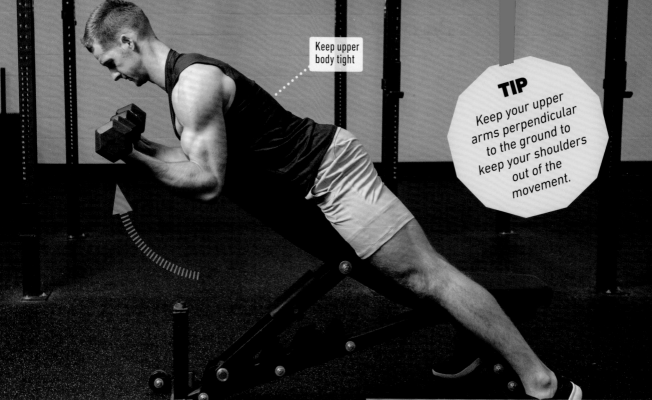

Keep upper body tight

TIP

Keep your upper arms perpendicular to the ground to keep your shoulders out of the movement.

[2] Using just the elbows as the hinge, pull the dumbbells upward using just your biceps. Pause briefly when you feel your biceps fully contract,

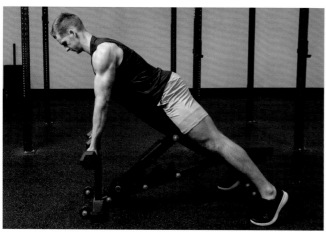

[3] Slowly lower the dumbbells back down to just above the starting position to keep tension in the muscle.

VARIATIONS

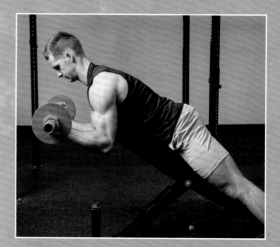

⬆ **EZ bar spider curl (easier)** Perform the exercise as you would with dumbbells. (The EZ bar allows for more stability and a variety of grip options.)

Spider curl on the preacher curl station Hold the dumbbells with a supinated grip and lean over the flat side of the preacher curl station. Place your upper arm against the angled side and perform the exercise. (This variation can help you better isolate the biceps.)

TARGETS /// triceps (primary); forearms (secondary)
EQUIPMENT /// bench and EZ bar

SKULLCRUSHERS

Don't let the name scare you—this exercise chisels the triceps! It also increases your strength for other presses. Though the standard movement targets the long head of the triceps, you can hit all three heads by changing grips, adjusting the bench angle, or changing the upper arm angle.

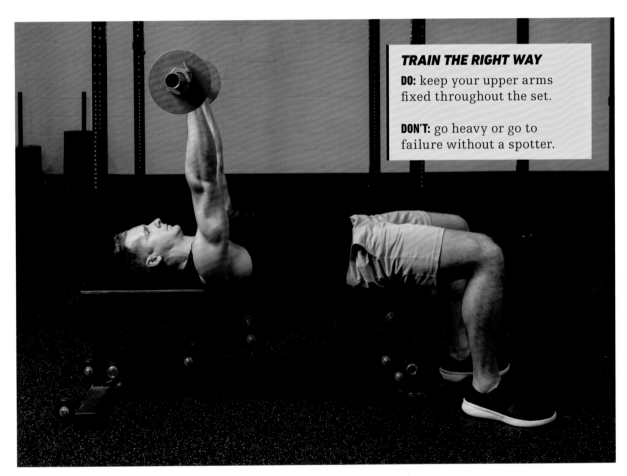

TRAIN THE RIGHT WAY

DO: keep your upper arms fixed throughout the set.

DON'T: go heavy or go to failure without a spotter.

[1] Sit on the end of the bench with your feet placed flat on the ground. Place the EZ bar in your lap and grasp the bar with an inside grip. Lie back on the bench while simultaneously extending the bar straight overhead.

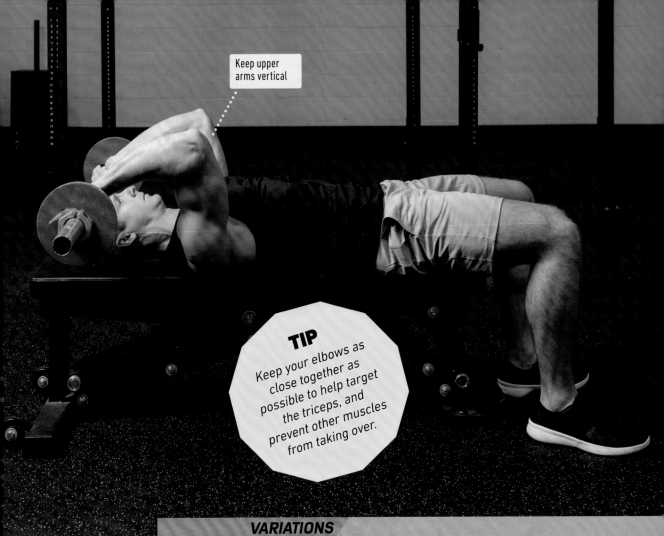

Keep upper arms vertical

TIP
Keep your elbows as close together as possible to help target the triceps, and prevent other muscles from taking over.

[2] Push your glutes into the bench, rotate your shoulders back and down, and hinge at the elbows to slowly lower the bar down until it's just above your forehead, pause, then push the bar back up to the starting position.

VARIATIONS

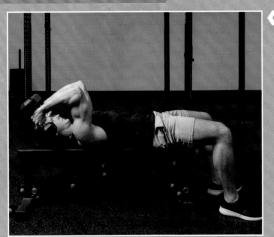

Dumbbell neutral-grip skullcrushers (more challenging) Perform the same movement using dumbbells. (This variation ensures that both sides are working evenly, and can help even out any asymmetries.)

Incline bench skullcrushers (more challenging) Adjust the bench to a 45-degree angle. Position your upper arms to be close to perpendicular to the ground, or slightly beyond. Extend through the elbow as you would with standard skullcrushers.

TARGETS /// triceps (primary); chest, lats (secondary)
EQUIPMENT /// high-pulley cable and v-bar attachment

TRICEPS PUSHDOWN

Build size and strength in your triceps by incorporating pushdowns into your program. This movement focuses on the long head of the triceps, which can tie the arms together beautifully with the back of the shoulders.

[1] Face the cable and grasp the v-bar with an overhand grip. Position your feet shoulder-width apart, keep your knees soft, and lean forward at a slight angle. Begin with the handle positioned at about chest-height.

Hinge at elbows

TIP
This exercise is commonly performed incorrectly, so stay focused during each rep and pay close attention to form to get maximum results.

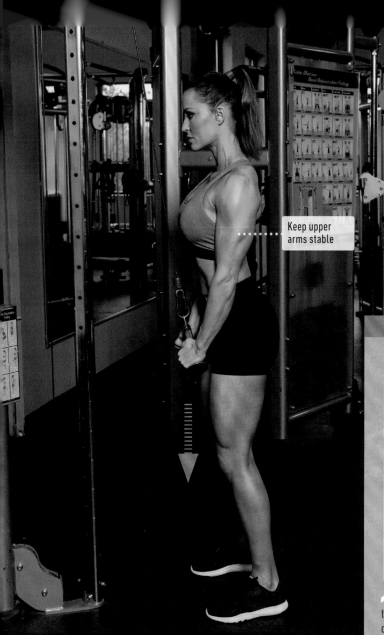

Keep upper
arms stable

TRAIN THE RIGHT WAY

DO: keep your upper body still
and keep your shoulders back.

DON'T: lean over the cable, as
this can cause your chest to
do more of the work.

VARIATIONS

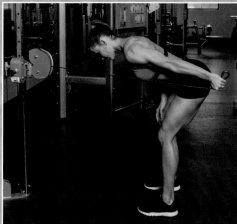

Kickbacks Lower the cable to chest height and use
the handle attachment, or grasp the ball portion of the
cable. Using a very light weight, grasp the cable with a
neutral grip and lean forward at the hips until the upper
body reaches almost parallel to the ground. Keeping your
upper arm by your side, extend the handle straight back
until your arm is fully extended.

Straight bar pushdown Attach a straight bar to a
high-pulley cable. Grasp the bar with an overhand grip
and perform the exercise as you would with the v-bar.
(You can adjust your grip width to target different areas
of the triceps. A wider grips tend to target the long and
medial heads of the triceps).

[2] With your elbows close to your body,
push the v-bar down until your arms are
fully extended, then slowly control the bar back
to the starting position.

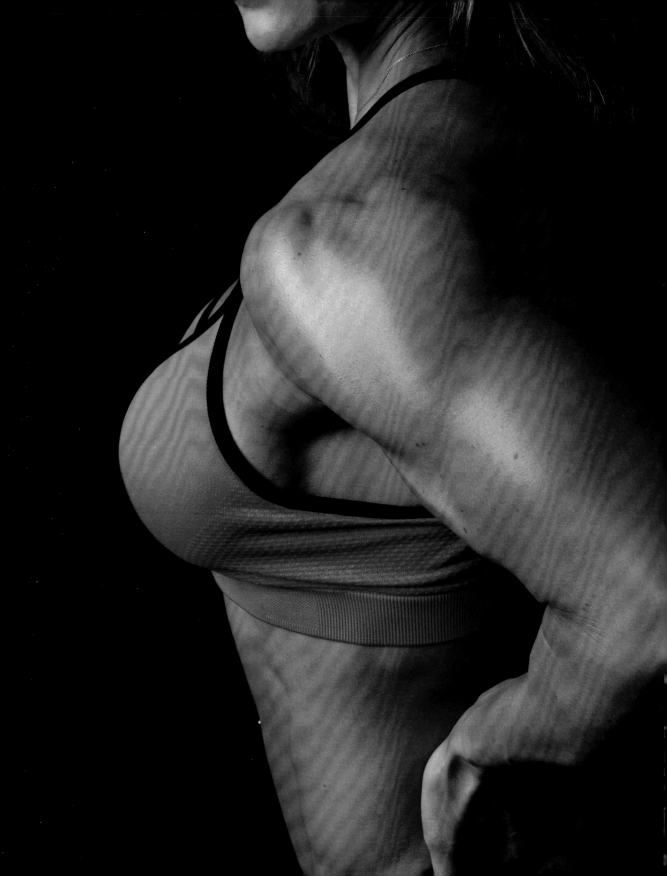

SHOULDERS

MILITARY PRESS

One of the six basic lifts, the military press has both aesthetic and functional benefits. Become proficient at pressing and you'll enjoy broad, beautiful shoulders, a strong core, and increased power. And increased power translates to better lifts and better jumping ability!

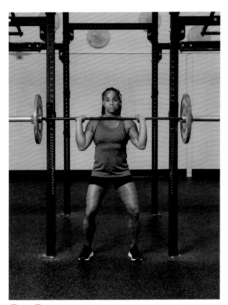

[1] Stand with your feet positioned shoulder-width apart and flat on the ground. Place your hands on the bar with an overhand grip that's slightly wider than shoulder-width apart, with your elbows positioned directly beneath your hands. Position the bar above your collarbone and keep your upper body leaning slightly back.

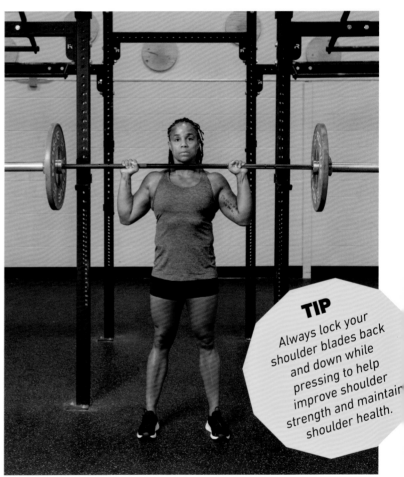

[2] Unrack the bar (stepping forward slightly if you're using a power rack) and hold the bar just above your collarbone.

TIP

Always lock your shoulder blades back and down while pressing to help improve shoulder strength and maintain shoulder health.

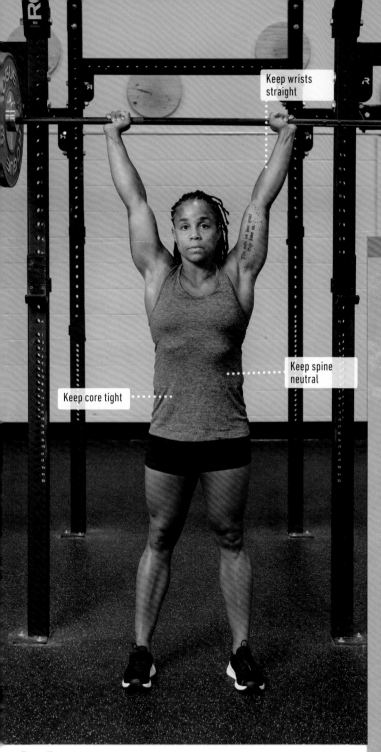

Keep wrists straight

Keep spine neutral

Keep core tight

TRAIN THE RIGHT WAY

DO: lean back as you lower the bar back down.

DON'T: push your head forward at full extension. (Your body should come forward.)

VARIATIONS

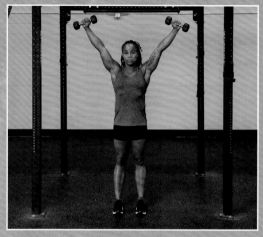

Narrow-to-wide press (more challenging) Choose dumbbells that are 50 to 60 percent of the weight you'd normally use. Start with an overhand grip and hold the dumbbells at shoulder-width. As you press, simultaneously push the dumbbells up and out.

Machine military press Adjust the machine seat to allow your upper arms to stop at parallel or just below. (This variation takes stabilizers out of the equation and also aids in going heavy without a spotter, so it's a great choice for building size and strength.)

Neutral-grip dumbbell press Hold dumbbells with your palms facing each other throughout the range of motion. (This variation better hits the medial head of the shoulders.)

Standing dumbbell military press Stand with your feet shoulder-width apart and on soft knees. Keep your back flat as you press. (Standing presses use more stabilizer muscles than seated presses.)

[3] Push the bar upward until your arms are fully extended (your upper body should come forward slightly as you press, and your arms should be in line with your ears at the full extension of the bar), pause, then lower the bar back down to the starting position.

TARGETS /// delts, traps (primary); forearms (secondary)
EQUIPMENT /// EZ bar and plates

WIDE-GRIP UPRIGHT ROW

Of all the upright row variations, the wide-grip upright row is the safest and most effective. It targets the side and rear delts, which creates width in the shoulders and makes the waist appear smaller. If you've tried upright rows in the past and found them uncomfortable, the wide-grip should feel better.

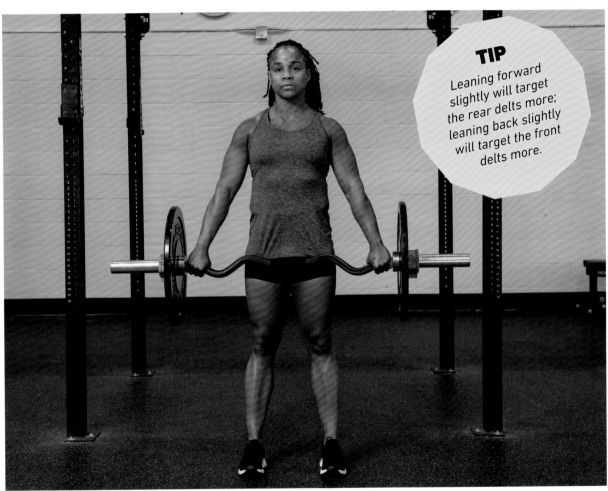

TIP
Leaning forward slightly will target the rear delts more; leaning back slightly will target the front delts more.

[1] Stand tall with your feet positioned shoulder-width apart. Hold the EZ bar with your arms extended downward, and with an overhand grip that's twice as wide as your shoulders.

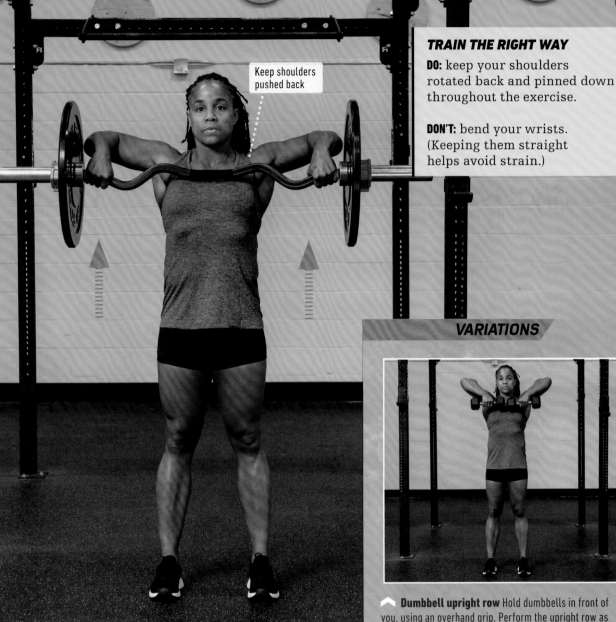

Keep shoulders
pushed back

TRAIN THE RIGHT WAY

DO: keep your shoulders rotated back and pinned down throughout the exercise.

DON'T: bend your wrists. (Keeping them straight helps avoid strain.)

VARIATIONS

Dumbbell upright row Hold dumbbells in front of you, using an overhand grip. Perform the upright row as instructed. (Dumbbells allow you to work both sides independently to balance out any asymmetries. This variation can also be better for lifters who may have existing wrist issues.)

Cable upright row (more challenging) Adjust the cable to the bottom pin and use the EZ bar attachment. Hold the bar with an overhand grip and stand close to the cable. Perform the upright row as you would with free weights. (Cables provide the benefit of constant tension, which can help with activating and building muscle.)

[2] Using your delts, pull the bar up to your chin, stopping just before your wrists bend, then slowly lower the bar back down to the starting position.

TARGETS **///** rear delts, upper lats (primary); forearms (secondary)
EQUIPMENT **///** adjustable bench, high-pulley cable, and rope attachment

INCLINE BENCH CABLE HIGH ROW

Rear delts finish the look of the upper back and create the perfect proportions, and while the set-up of this exercise requires a few steps, the extra effort will be rewarded with more highly defined rear delts.

[1] Adjust the bench to a 60- to 70-degree incline, and position it so that the low end of the bench is facing the cable pulley and the front of the bench is 1 to 2 feet [.3m to .6m] away from the cable). Adjust the cable to the highest pin and secure the rope attachment. Grasp the rope using an overhand grip, and sit with your back against the bench. Extend your arms to form a straight line with the cable.

TIP
Opt for a lighter weight to help you better isolate the rear delts on each rep.

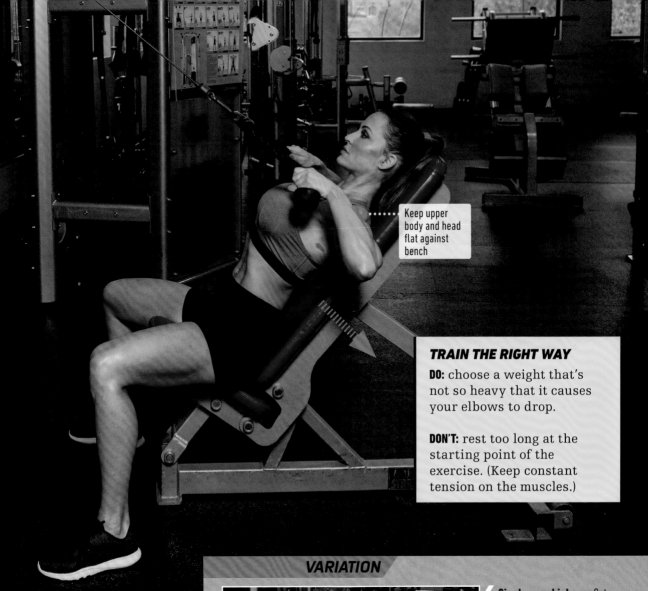

Keep upper body and head flat against bench

TRAIN THE RIGHT WAY

DO: choose a weight that's not so heavy that it causes your elbows to drop.

DON'T: rest too long at the starting point of the exercise. (Keep constant tension on the muscles.)

[2] Keeping your elbows high, pull the rope to about chin level while squeezing your shoulder blades together at mid-rep, then control the rope back to the starting point.

VARIATION

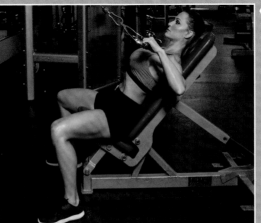

❮ **Single-arm high row** Set the bench up as you would for the double-arm exercise and attach the handle to the cable. Grasp the handle and pull it to chin level, while keeping your elbow high. Start with your nondominant side, then perform on the opposite side while repeating the same number of reps. (This variation can help eliminate muscle imbalances.)

TARGETS /// rear delts, rhomboids (primary); lats, traps (secondary)
EQUIPMENT /// cable pulley and rope attachment

HIGH ROW

The rear delts are a small muscle and can be tough to isolate, but well-defined rear delts can balance the shoulders and add the perfect amount of width to the upper body. Find the sweet spot between strength and finesse with this exercise, and you will see great results!

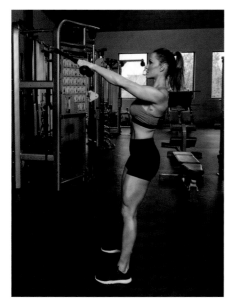

[1] Adjust the cable to the top pin. Stand with your feet shoulder-width apart and with a slight bend in your knees. Grasp the rope attachment with an overhand grip and keep your arms extended.

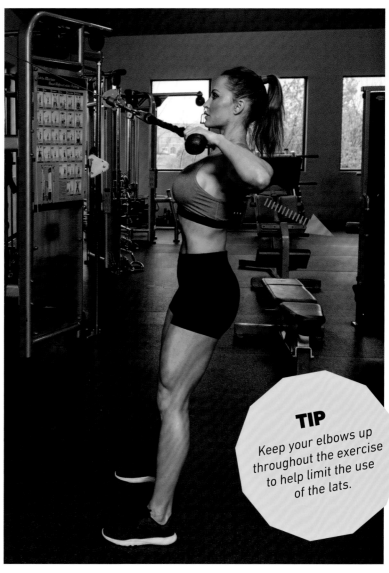

TIP
Keep your elbows up throughout the exercise to help limit the use of the lats.

[2] Pull the rope straight back toward your chin while simultaneously rotating your forearms up and slightly outward.

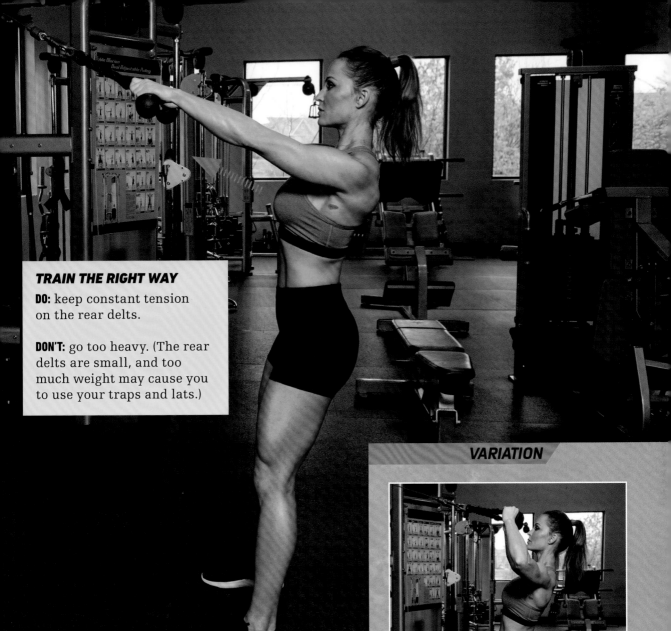

TRAIN THE RIGHT WAY

DO: keep constant tension on the rear delts.

DON'T: go too heavy. (The rear delts are small, and too much weight may cause you to use your traps and lats.)

VARIATION

[**3**] Pause momentarily when your hands reach your chin, then slowly release the rope back to the starting position while rotating your hands and arms back to their original positions.

High row with external rotation Use a weight slightly lighter than you would normally use for the high row. Pull the rope to your chin and rotate your forearms upward and backward until you feel a good stretch.

LATERAL RAISE

Well-developed side delts can add width and shape to the upper body, so if you want round and full "caps," the side delts are the muscles to train. Strong side delts also can improve pressing power, and the lateral raise does an excellent job of targeting these muscles.

TIP
This muscle is small, so choose a weight that's heavy enough to stress the side delt, but not so heavy that stronger surrounding muscles take over.

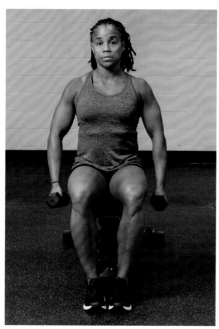

[1] Sit on a bench with your upper body tall and feet flat on the ground. Hold the dumbbells at your sides, using a neutral overhand grip, with your thumbs tilted slightly inward. Bend your arms just slightly.

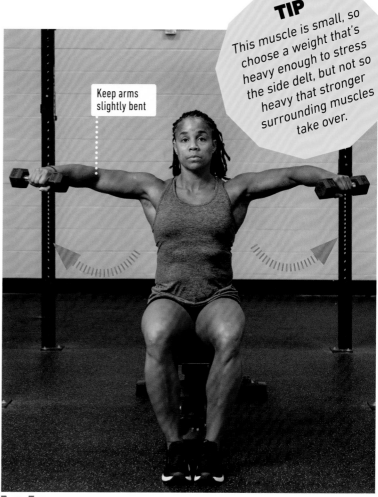

Keep arms slightly bent

[2] "Push" the dumbbells away from your body in an arc until your upper arms are just above parallel to the ground, pausing at the top of the rep.

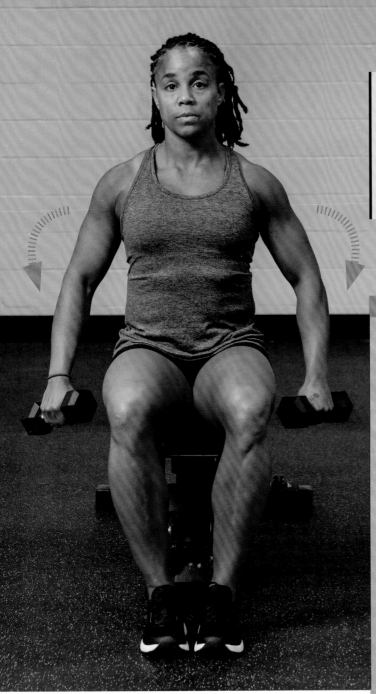

TRAIN THE RIGHT WAY

DO: lead the exercise with pinky fingers and keep the elbows tilted up slightly.

DON'T: bounce or shrug the weight before you perform the raise.

VARIATIONS

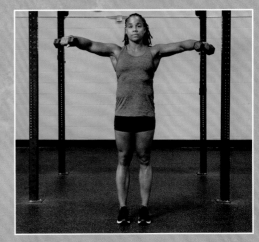

Standing lateral raise (easier) Perform these just as you would the seated version, but while standing on soft knees. (Don't use momentum to swing the weight.)

Single-arm cable raise (more challenging) Adjust the cable to the bottom pin and use a handle attachment. Stand perpendicular to the machine and grasp the handle with your outside hand. Perform the raise just as you would with the dumbbells. (Cables provide constant tension, which aids muscle growth.)

Machine lateral raise (easier) Adjust the seat to the proper height and place your elbows under the pads. Pin your shoulder blades back and down, and perform the raises.

[3] Slowly lower the weight back down to just above the starting point.

TARGETS /// rear and side delts, rhomboids, traps (primary); upper lats (secondary)
EQUIPMENT /// adjustable bench and dumbbells

REVERSE FLYE

Many shoulder and chest exercises develop the front delts well, but can leave the side and rear delts lacking development. Not only can the reverse flye build more complete shoulders, but it can also develop better overall symmetry, improve posture, and increase your strength for other lifts.

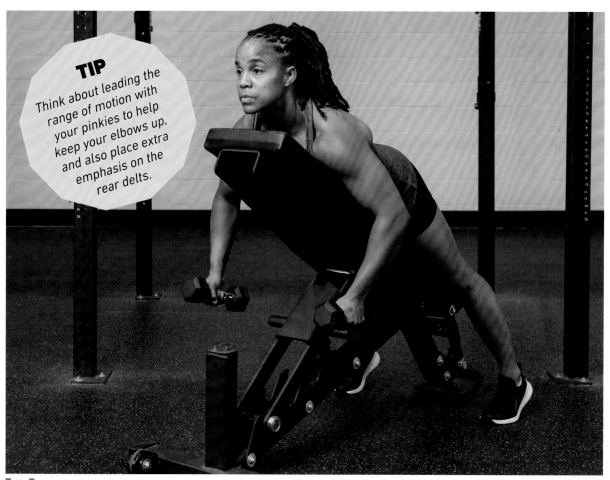

TIP
Think about leading the range of motion with your pinkies to help keep your elbows up, and also place extra emphasis on the rear delts.

[1] Adjust the bench to a 60-degree angle. Grasp a pair of dumbbells with a neutral grip and lie stomach-down on the bench with your feet placed firmly on the ground. Extend the dumbbells down toward the ground.

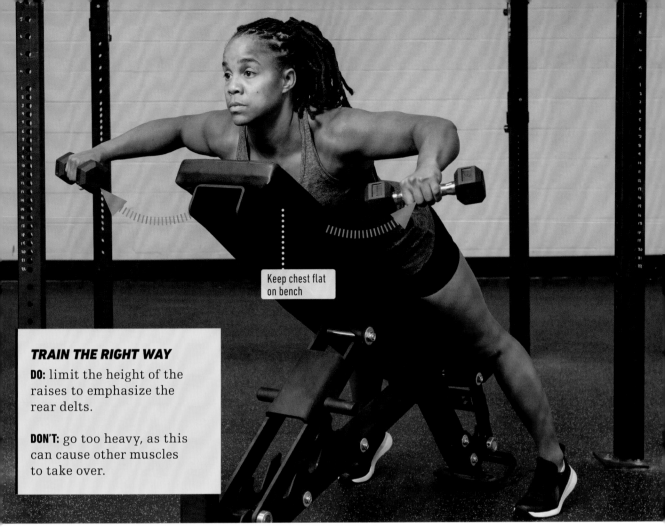

Keep chest flat on bench

TRAIN THE RIGHT WAY

DO: limit the height of the raises to emphasize the rear delts.

DON'T: go too heavy, as this can cause other muscles to take over.

[2] With a slight bend in the elbows, raise the dumbbells upward and outward in an arc until your upper arms reach parallel, pause, then slowly lower the dumbbells back down until just before the starting point.

VARIATIONS

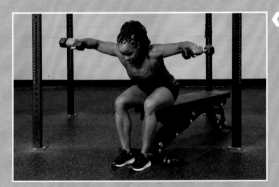

Seated reverse flye Sit on a bench and hold two dumbbells with a neutral grip. Lean forward until your upper body is at a 45-degree angle. (If possible, lower yourself all the way down until your chest is resting on your knees.) Position the dumbbells just behind your heels. Perform the exercise as you would on the incline bench.

Reverse cable flye (more challenging) Adjust two cable pulleys to about shoulder height and secure a handle attachment to each side. With an overhand grip, reach across your body and grab one handle, then do the same on the opposite side. Press the cables out in front of you, making sure they are crossed, and perform the flyes as you would normally.

FRONT RAISE

Well-developed front delts add fullness to the upper body and tie the shoulders into the chest, while adding shoulder stability and improving strength to help reduce the chance of injury.

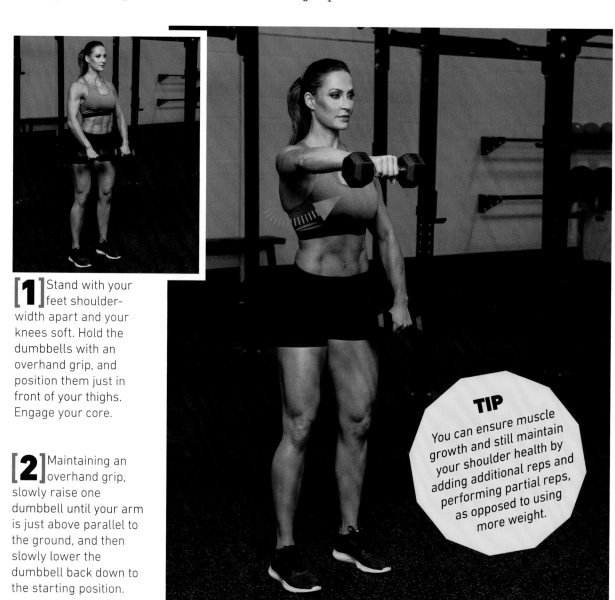

[1] Stand with your feet shoulder-width apart and your knees soft. Hold the dumbbells with an overhand grip, and position them just in front of your thighs. Engage your core.

[2] Maintaining an overhand grip, slowly raise one dumbbell until your arm is just above parallel to the ground, and then slowly lower the dumbbell back down to the starting position.

TIP
You can ensure muscle growth and still maintain your shoulder health by adding additional reps and performing partial reps, as opposed to using more weight.

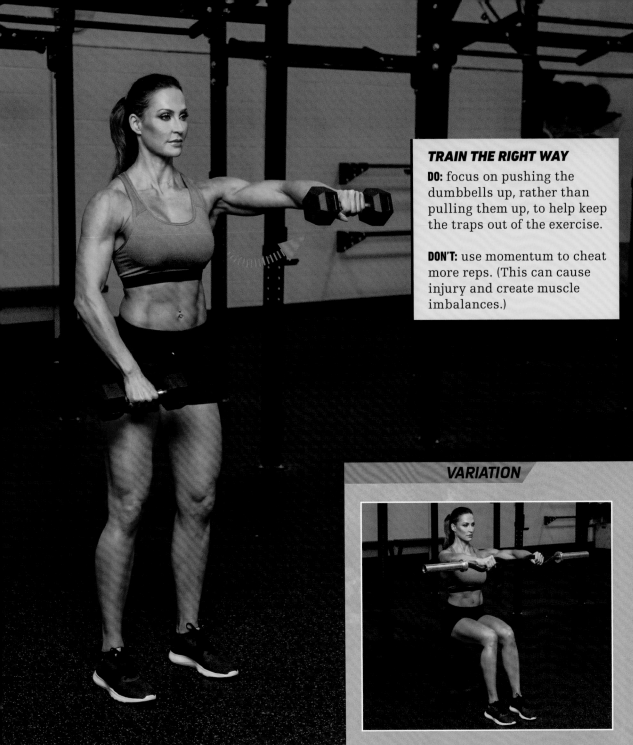

VARIATION

Seated EZ bar partial front raise Sit on a half bench and hold an EZ bar with an overhand grip. Extend your arms forward until the bar is near your knees. Raise the bar to just above parallel and lower the bar down until it almost touches your knees. (This variation is a great finisher.)

[3] Repeat the movement on the opposite side, continuing to alternate reps on each side.

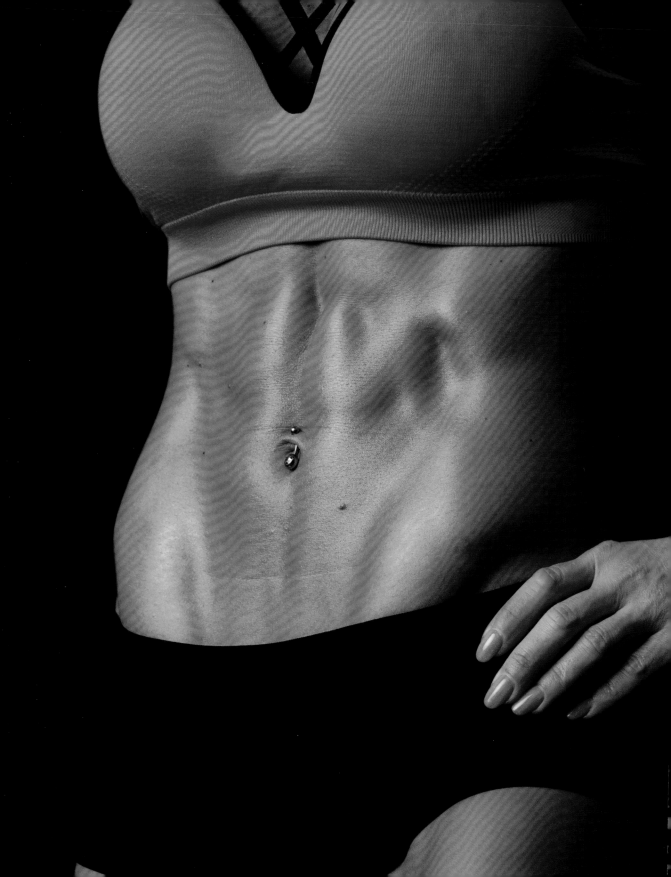

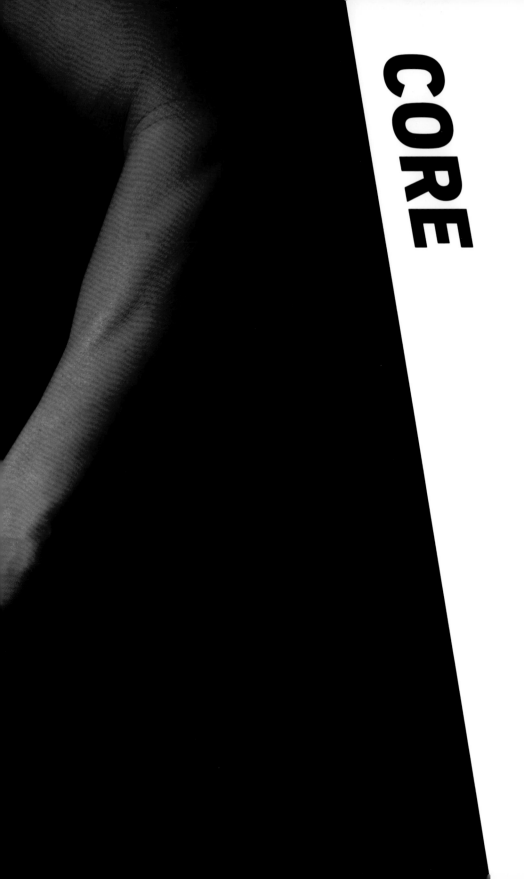

CORE

TARGETS /// abs, obliques, lats (primary); lower back, chest (secondary)
EQUIPMENT /// medicine ball

MEDICINE BALL SLAMS

Though the main focus of medicine ball slams is to develop strong abs, it also can help increase overall power. It's a great whole body exercise that can improve the flow of your physique, burn tons of calories, and improve hand-eye coordination.

VARIATION

Oblique throws Stand with one side to a wall or a partner. Keeping your feet flat, rotate at the hips to extend the medicine ball behind your body, then forcefully rotate at the hips to throw the ball across your body as hard as possible. Repeat on both sides. (This better targets the obliques.)

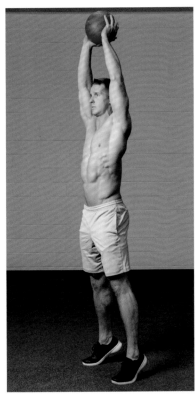

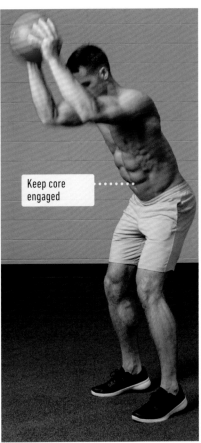

Keep core engaged

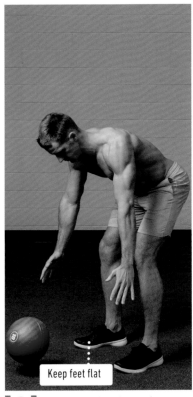

Keep feet flat

[1] Position your feet shoulder-width apart, and hold the medicine ball straight above your head with your arms extended. Engage your core and rise up on your toes.

[2] Keeping your feet anchored, engage your core and lats and bend forward at the waist as you forcefully throw the medicine ball against the ground with as much force as possible.

[3] Complete the throw bent at the waist and with your arms extended. Pick up the ball and repeat.

TARGETS /// inner abs, abs (primary); obliques (secondary)
EQUIPMENT /// none

VACUUM

The vacuum is the most effective exercise for tightening the midsection and decreasing its diameter. It also improves overall abdominal control, which can translate to stronger lifts and a reduced chance of injury.

VARIATION

Lying vacuum (easier) Lie flat on your back with your pelvis rolled forward, knees bent, and feet flat on the ground. Perform the vacuum as you would standing.

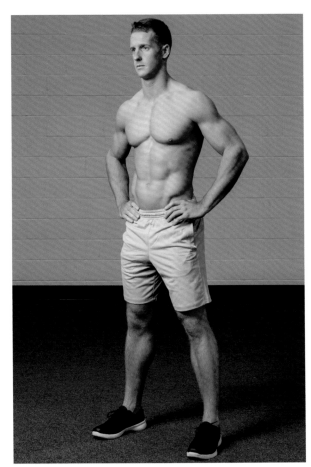

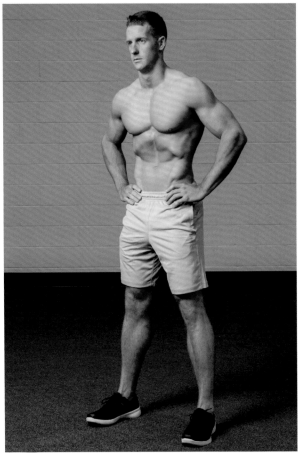

[1] Stand tall with your hands on your hips, and your feet positioned shoulder-width apart.

[2] Exhale all the air from your lungs and hold your breath, while simultaneously expanding your ribcage and pulling your belly button upward and inward. Hold for a minimum of 10 seconds, or up to 30 seconds.

TARGETS **///** obliques, abs (primary); lats, chest (secondary)
EQUIPMENT **///** high-pulley cable with handle attachment

CABLE CHOP

When you think about abs exercises, crunches, or other floor exercises usually
come to mind. But some of the most effective abs exercises are performed
while standing. The cable chop can chisel your midsection, and also help
protect your back for everyday activities like golfing or lifting heavy objects.

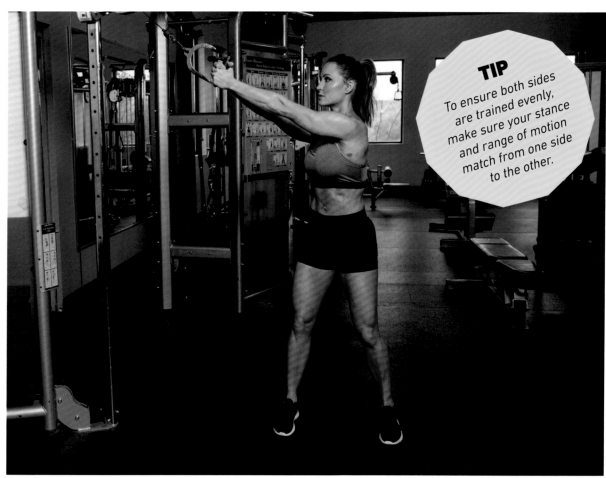

TIP
To ensure both sides
are trained evenly,
make sure your stance
and range of motion
match from one side
to the other.

[1] Adjust the cable pulley to the highest pin and attach the handle. Stand with
one side to the cable, with your feet positioned about twice the width of
your shoulders. Extend your arms and grasp the handle with both hands, using
an overlapping grip, and then take a side step away from the machine to create
tension on the cable.

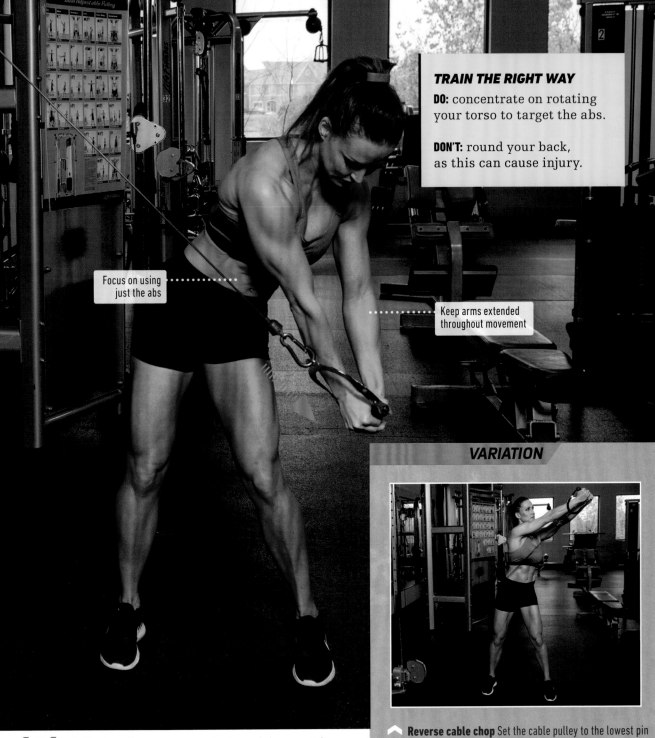

Focus on using just the abs

Keep arms extended throughout movement

VARIATION

Reverse cable chop Set the cable pulley to the lowest pin and simply reverse the movement for the exercise, "chopping" from low to high. (This variation works the abs and obliques, along with the shoulders.)

[2] Pull the handle across your body and downward until the handle reaches your opposite knee, then slowly control the weight back to the starting point.

KNEE-UPS

Toning the lower abs can be a challenge for many people. While it's technically not possible to spot reduce, it is possible to strengthen underlying muscles and create a firmer look. This exercise is particularly effective at strengthening and tightening the lower abs to help increase definition.

[1] Stand facing away from a dip chair or dip station. Place your back against the backrest, place your forearms on the pads (if using a dip chair), and grasp the handles. Allow your legs to dangle straight down.

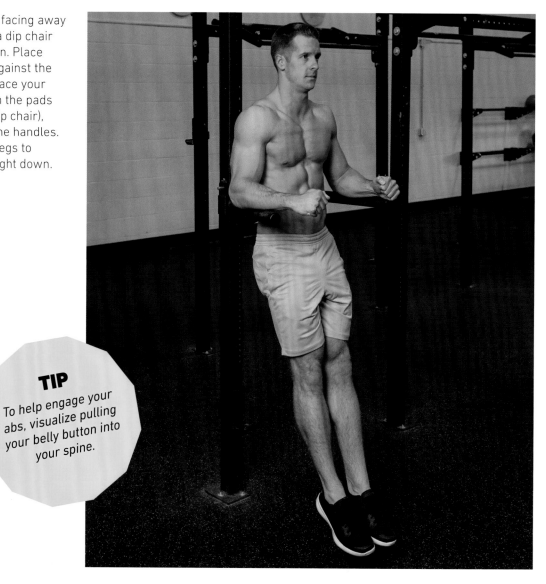

TIP
To help engage your abs, visualize pulling your belly button into your spine.

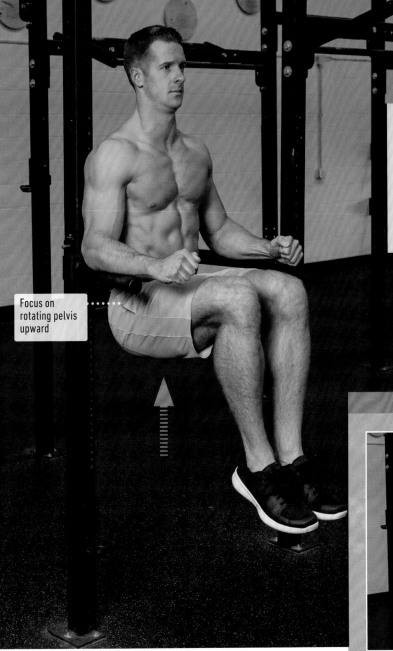

Focus on rotating pelvis upward

TRAIN THE RIGHT WAY

DO: move slowly, and focus on feeling your abs contract.

DON'T: use momentum. (This can tweak your lower back and cause other muscles to take over.)

[2] Engage your core and slowly lift your knees up toward your chest until your upper leg reaches parallel to the ground, then slowly lower your legs back down to the starting position.

VARIATIONS

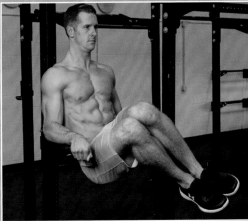

Side raises Lift your knees upward while simultaneously rotating your legs to one side until your lower legs reach about parallel. then lower your legs back down to the starting position. Repeat on the opposite side. (This variation better targets the obliques.)

L-ups (more challenging) Keeping your legs straight, hinge at the hips and slowly raise your legs up until they reach parallel to the ground, then slowly lower them back down to the starting position.

TARGETS *III* inner abs, abs, lower back (primary); shoulders (secondary)
EQUIPMENT *III* yoga mat

PLANK

It's important to not only work the surface muscles
of the abs, but the underlying muscles, as well.
The plank is the perfect exercise for targeting all
of those core muscles, including the transverse
abdominus, or TVA, which acts as an internal
girdle to provide stability for heavy lifts, and
also can create the look of a smaller waist.

VARIATION

Side plank Perform on your side, while
propped up on one forearm and on the
outer edge of one foot. Your body should be
aligned from head to toes, and your
opposite hand should be placed on your hip.
Repeat on the opposite side. (This variation
better targets the obliques.)

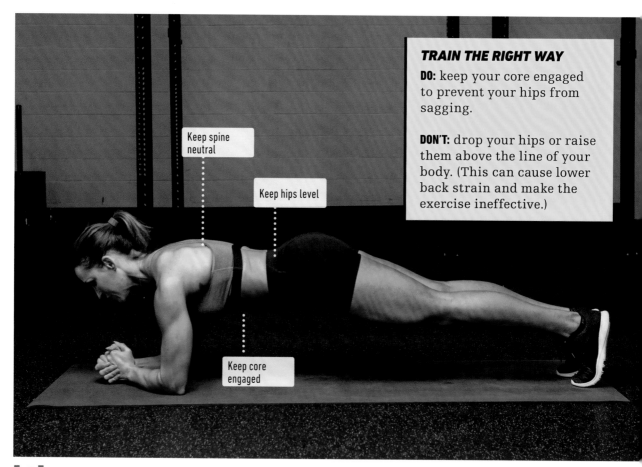

TRAIN THE RIGHT WAY

DO: keep your core engaged
to prevent your hips from
sagging.

DON'T: drop your hips or raise
them above the line of your
body. (This can cause lower
back strain and make the
exercise ineffective.)

Keep spine
neutral

Keep hips level

Keep core
engaged

[1] Begin stomach-down on the mat. Prop yourself up onto your forearms,
clasp your hands, and rise up onto your toes to form a straight line from
your head to your heels. Hold.

TARGETS *III* abs, hip flexors, transverse abdominis (primary); quads, glutes (secondary)
EQUIPMENT *III* yoga mat

FLUTTER KICKS

A good strength training program borrows effective training techniques from all disciplines to create a well-rounded physique. Swimmers are known for their toned and streamlined bodies, and flutter kicks emulate the kicking movement that gives aquatic athletes those tight abs.

VARIATION

Scissor kicks Rather that kicking your legs up and down, lift them off the ground and kick outward and inward, crossing your legs in the middle and alternating between moving your left foot and right foot on top each time your legs cross.

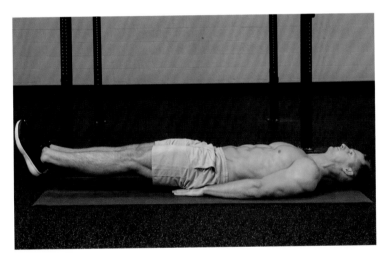

[1] Lie flat on your back with your hands tucked under your glutes. Engage your core and lift your legs slightly off the ground, with your toes pointed.

[2] Keepng your knees straight, begin making a fluttering motion with your legs by alternately kicking one leg upward about 1 foot (30.5cm) off the ground, then kicking the opposite leg upward. Repeat in a rapid, continuous motion.

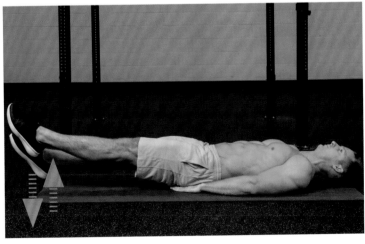

TARGETS /// obliques, abs (primary); hip flexors (secondary)
EQUIPMENT /// yoga mat

V-UP

This bodyweight exercise effectively targets every muscle in the abs. It requires good upper- and lower-body coordination and proper timing to execute, but it will help you create more defined abs, a stronger core, and better balance.

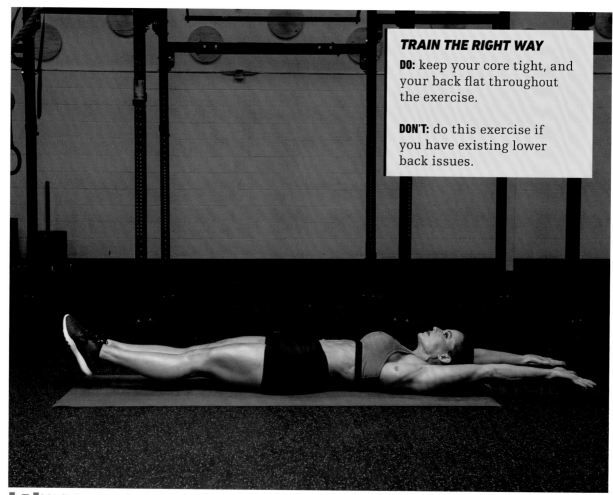

TRAIN THE RIGHT WAY

DO: keep your core tight, and your back flat throughout the exercise.

DON'T: do this exercise if you have existing lower back issues.

[1] Lie flat on your back, extend your arms straight over your head, and extend your legs straight out with your toes pointed. Lift your arms and legs slightly off the ground.

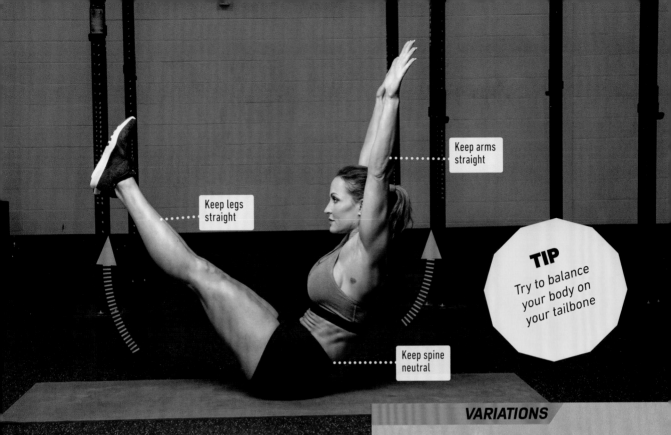

Keep arms straight

Keep legs straight

Keep spine neutral

TIP
Try to balance your body on your tailbone

[2] With a tight core, simultaneously lift your legs and upper body off the ground to form a "v" shape at mid-rep.

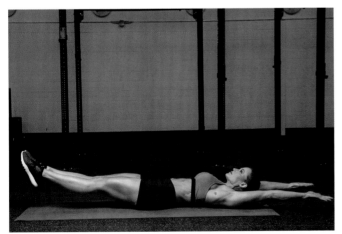

[3] In a controlled fashion, lower your upper body and legs back down to the starting position.

VARIATIONS

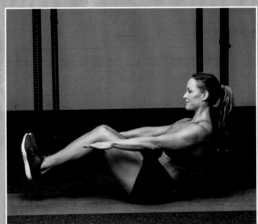

Tuck-up (easier) Rather than keeping your legs extended, pull your knees toward your chest and keep your arms parallel to the ground. (This variation is better for beginners.)

Lying L-up (easier) Lie flat on your back and tuck your hands under your hips. Extend your legs straight out and raise them up until they're perpendicular to the ground.

TARGETS **///** obliques, abs, inner abs (primary); shoulders, lower back (secondary)
EQUIPMENT **///** yoga mat

RUSSIAN TWIST

You'll make your obliques pop and strengthen your core with this exercise. This move is more challenging than it looks, as you'll be working to pull your abs in, while simultaneously stabilizing your body and twisting. Begin with just your body weight and advance to weights as you become more proficient.

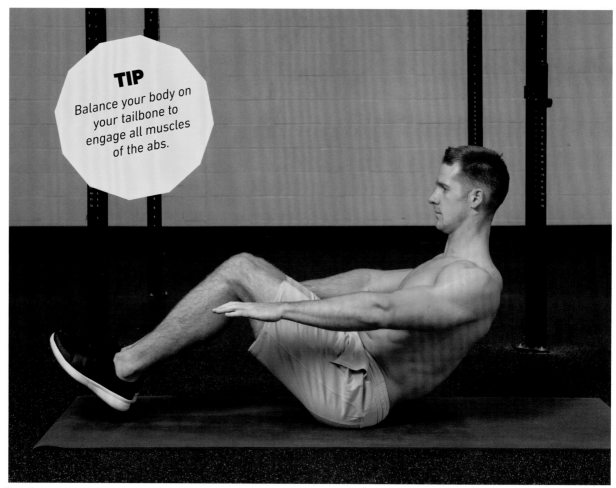

TIP
Balance your body on your tailbone to engage all muscles of the abs.

[1] From a seated position, bend your knees, lean back until your upper body reaches a 45-degree angle, extend your arms straight out in front of you, and lift your feet slightly off the ground.

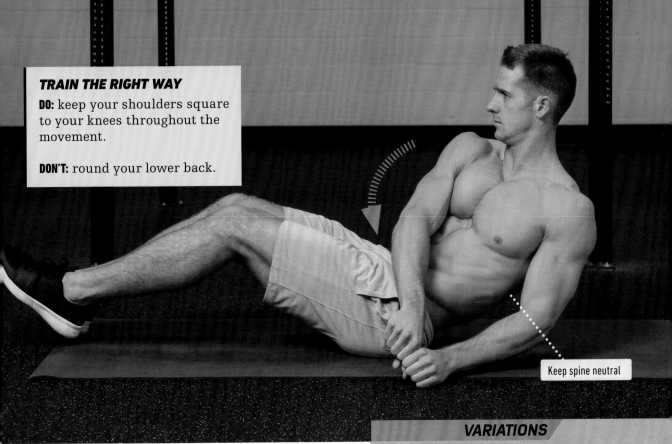

TRAIN THE RIGHT WAY

DO: keep your shoulders square to your knees throughout the movement.

DON'T: round your lower back.

Keep spine neutral

[2] Rotate your arms to one side until you feel your upper body begin to twist.

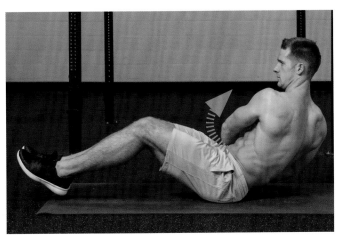

[3] Slowly rotate your arms over to the opposite side. Repeat the movement from side to side in a continuous motion.

VARIATIONS

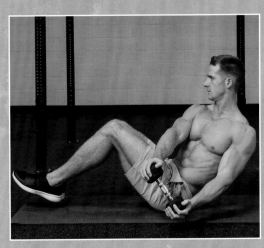

⌃ Weighted Russian twist (more challenging)
Perform the exercise holding a small plate, medicine ball, or dumbbell.

Russian twist on a decline bench (more challenging)
Secure your feet under the pad and sit back. Keep your upper body tall and perform the exercise as instructed. (This variation targets more of the lower abs.)

REVERSE CRUNCH

Attaining a "six pack" requires training both the upper and lower sections of the rectus abdominis. And while defining the upper sections can be achieved through a clean diet and indirect abs training, the lower sections often need more direct work. The reverse crunch can produce this result through constant tension.

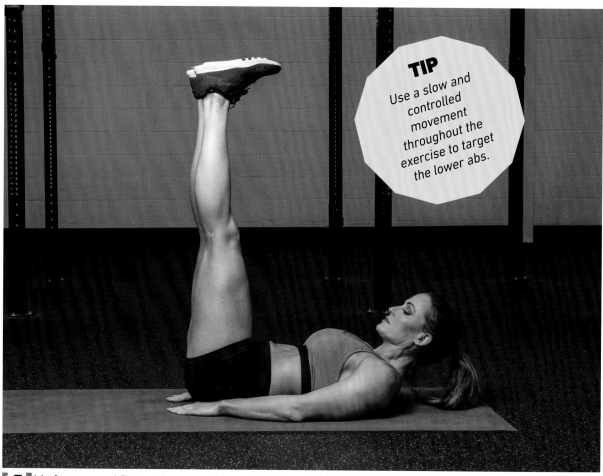

TIP
Use a slow and controlled movement throughout the exercise to target the lower abs.

[1] Lie face up and flat on the ground. Place both hands alongside your hips, with palms facing down. Lift your legs up until they're perpendicular to the ground.

VARIATION

▲ **Reverse crunch against a wall (more challenging)** Lie face up on the ground with your hips about 6 inches (15cm) from a wall, and your legs straight and parallel to the wall. Lift your hips off the ground, using the wall to keep your legs straight.

[2] Using your lower abs, slowly lift your hips straight up and off the floor, keeping your legs straight, and your hands at your hips while using your arms to keep your body anchored. Slowly lower your hips back down to the starting position.

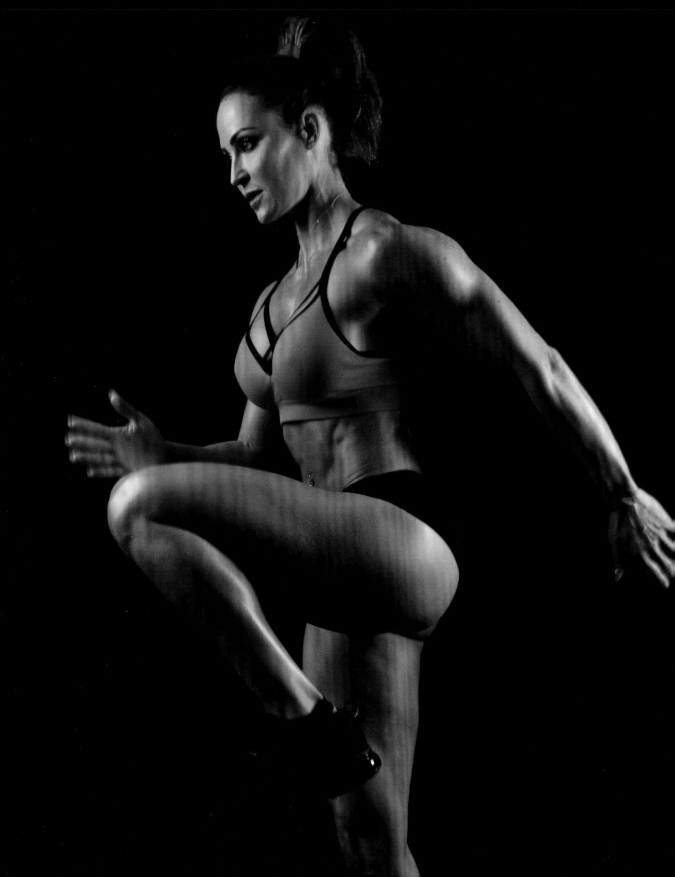

CARDIO

BURPEE

The burpee is the ultimate do-anywhere, total body exercise that will develop strength, power, and a strong core. Burpees fit into almost training program and can be used as a finisher, a standalone workout, or as part of a HIIT circuit.

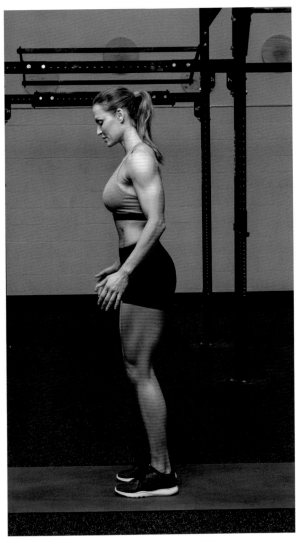

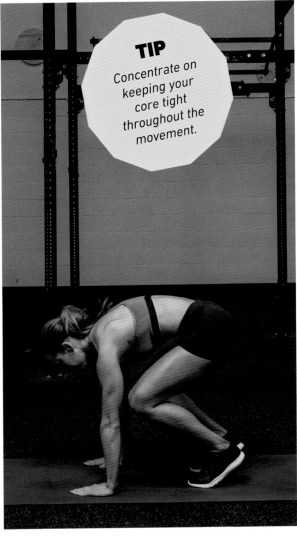

TIP
Concentrate on keeping your core tight throughout the movement.

[1] Begin in a standing position with your hands at your sides.

[2] Crouch down and place your hands flat on the ground in front of you.

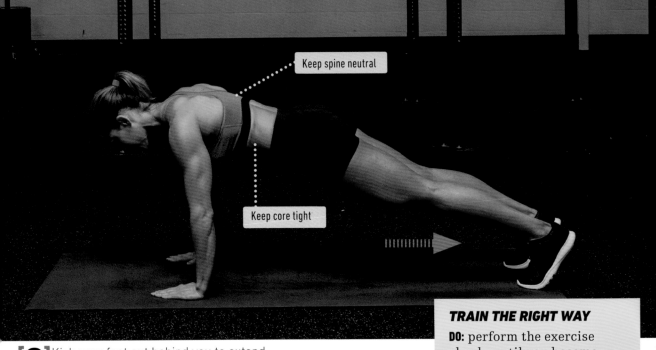

Keep spine neutral

Keep core tight

[3] Kick your feet out behind you to extend into a high plank position.

TRAIN THE RIGHT WAY

DO: perform the exercise slowly until you become proficient at it.

DON'T: round your back, or let your hips sag while in the plank position.

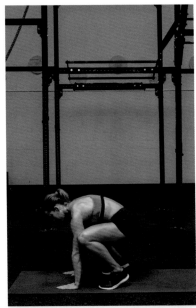

[4] Keeping your hands flat on the ground, jump your feet back to your hands.

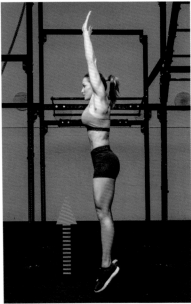

[5] Explosively jump straight up while extending your hands straight above your head before landing back in the starting position.

VARIATIONS

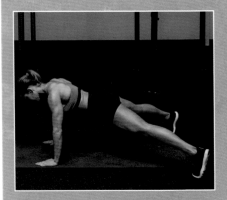

Burpee jack (more challenging) Kick both legs out as if you were doing a jumping jack, then kick both legs back in.

Burpee with a push-up (more challenging) Perform a push-up after dropping into the plank.

HIGH KNEES

Sprints are one of the quickest ways to elevate the heart rate and train the entire body, but full sprints can be very taxing on the body. High knees allow you to train anywhere and reap the benefits of sprints without affecting your recovery.

VARIATION

High knees march (easier) Instead of a sprint, perform the exercise slowly, squeezing the opposite hamstring and glute with each leg drive. (This variation is great for glute activation.)

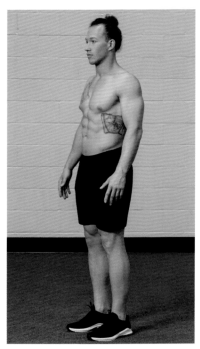

[1] Stand with your feet shoulder-width apart and your arms at your sides.

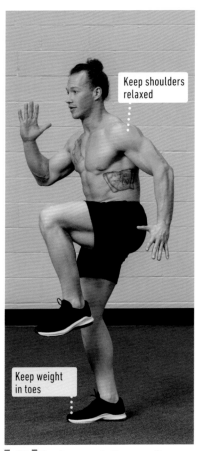

Keep shoulders relaxed

Keep weight in toes

[2] Begin a sprinting motion by driving one knee upward until the upper leg reaches parallel to the ground while swinging your opposing arm forward and up.

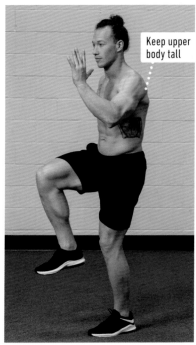

Keep upper body tall

[3] Repeat the movement with the opposite arm and leg. Repeat the movement in a rapid, continuous fashion to perform a sprint in place.

TARGETS *///* quads, glutes, hamstrings (primary); hip flexors, abs (secondary)
EQUIPMENT *///* none

SPEED SKATER

Olympic speed skaters are known for their powerful legs. By emulating their workouts, you'll be able to sculpt your legs and also get a great cardio workout. (Performing unfamiliar exercises like this one helps stress the muscles to cause adaptations and growth.)

VARIATION

Skater lunge (easier) Rather than jumping, step from side to side, placing your weight evenly on both legs and performing a lunge on each side.

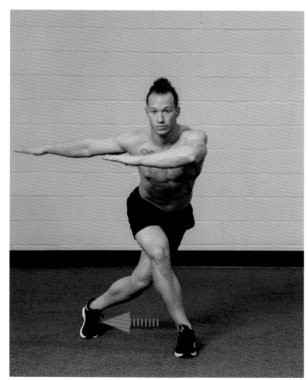

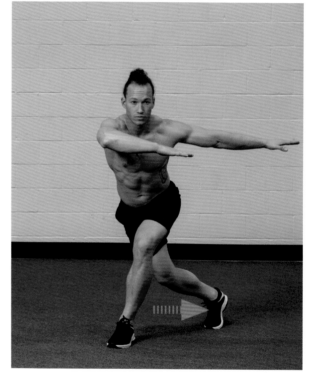

[1] Begin in a standing position with your arms at your sides and your feet positioned at shoulder width. Squat down to load your legs, and then push from your left leg to hop laterally to your right, landing in a quarter-squat position while simultaneously swinging your left leg behind your right, swinging your left arm forward and swinging your right arm to the side.

[2] Immediately push from your right leg to jump laterally to the left and landing on the left leg in a quarter-squat position while simultaneously swinging your right leg behind your left, and swinging your right arm forward and your left arm to the side. Repeat the movement in a back-and-forth, fluid motion.

TARGETS /// calves, quads, shoulders (primary); abs (secondary)
EQUIPMENT /// none

JUMPING JACK

You can get a cardio workout, improve your core stability, and train anywhere with this bodyweight classic. Use jumping jacks as a warm-up to improve circulation, or as a finisher in a circuit. The dynamic motion of this movement can help improve flexibility, as well.

VARIATION

Star jack (more challenging) Jump up higher than a normal jack, while simultaneously swinging your arms and kicking your legs out to the sides, then pulling your feet back in before landing.

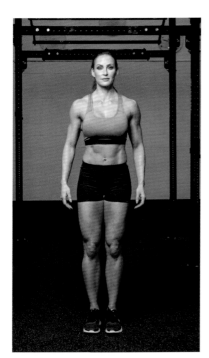

[1] Stand with your feet together and your arms at your sides.

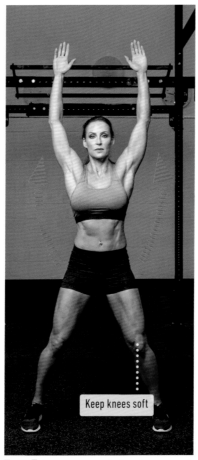

Keep knees soft

[2] Jump up and simultaneously widen your stance to about 1.5 times shoulder width, while swinging your arms out and over your head.

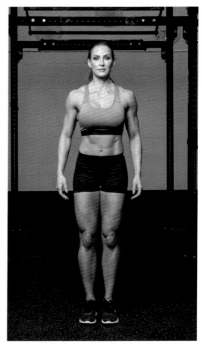

[3] Immediately jump again and bring your feet back together while lowering your arms back down to your sides. Repeat in a rapid, continuous motion.

TARGETS /// hamstrings, glutes, quads (primary); shoulders, abs (secondary)
EQUIPMENT /// none

SWITCH LUNGE

Light plyometric exercises activate fast twitch muscles, which are rounder and fuller-looking than slow twitch muscles. They also have a greater potential for growth, so if you're looking to sculpt your physique, explosive movements like the switch lunge can be beneficial.

VARIATION

Lunge jump (more challenging) Start in a full lunge position. Jump straight up, switch legs in mid-air, then land back in a full lunge. (Keep the reps to 10 or less.)

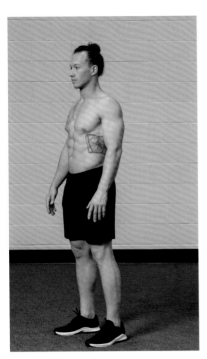

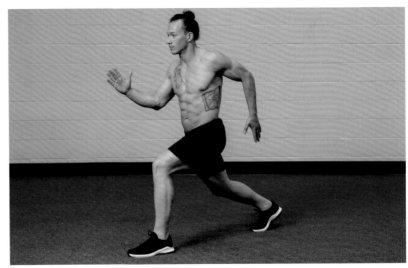

[1] Begin in a standing position with your feet positioned shoulder-width apart.

[2] Jump straight up and into a quarter-lunge position by jumping one leg forward while jumping the opposite leg back, and swinging the opposing arm forward and up, while swinging the other arm back.

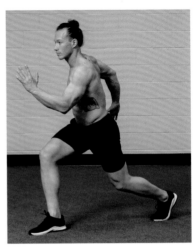

[3] Jump straight up and switch leg positions while simultaneously switching arm positions. Repeat in a rapid, continuous motion.

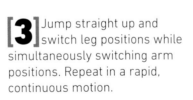

TARGETS /// glutes, hamstrings, quads (primary); calves (secondary)
EQUIPMENT /// none

POP SQUAT

This is another great exercise to work those fast twitch muscles. This move helps improve coordination and balance, and is a bit different than normal jump squats.

VARIATION

Jump squat (more challenging) From a squat position, explode upward using both your legs and your arms, and then softly land back in the squat position. (Keep the reps to 10 or less.)

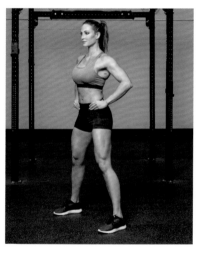

[1] Begin in a standing position with your feet wider than shoulder-width apart, and your hands on your hips.

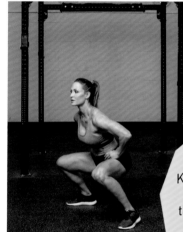

[2] Lower your body down until your upper legs are parallel with the ground.

TIP

Keep the squats shallow and push your weight through your toes to train the quads, or squat deeper with your weight through your heels to hit the glutes.

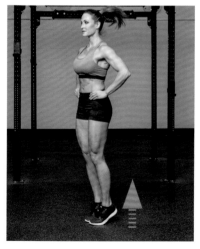

[3] Jump (or "pop") up out of the squat and land standing straight up, with your feet together.

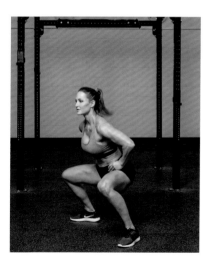

[4] Quickly jump straight up again and land back down in the squat position.

DYNAMIC STEP-UPS

Explosive, athletic bodyweight movements like dynamic step-ups help tie muscle groups together and create an aesthetic flow in the body. These are a favorite of track and field athletes for improving speed and power.

VARIATION

Beginner dynamic step-ups (easier)
Perform the exercise as instructed, but keep most of your body weight on the rear (down) leg.

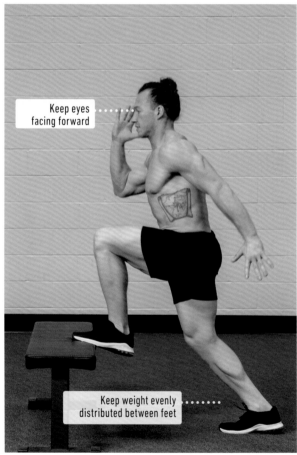

Keep eyes facing forward

Keep weight evenly distributed between feet

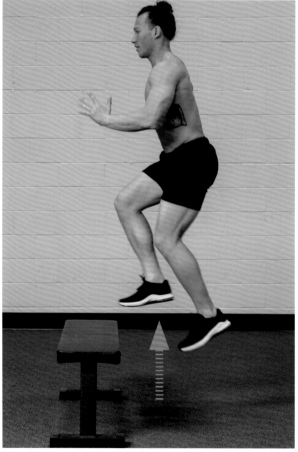

[1] Place one foot on the bench and one on the floor. Raise the arm opposite the raised leg forward, while pulling the opposing arm back.

[2] Jump up by simultaneously pushing off both feet, switching legs mid-jump, and landing with the opposite foot on the bench and opposite arm forward. Repeat in a continuous motion, switching arm and leg positions with each jump.

PLYO PUSH-UP

One of the best ways to improve upper-body power is to work against your own body weight. Using explosive moves like the plyo push-up will help you improve muscle fiber recruitment and enjoy gains in muscularity and strength.

[1] Lower your body down into a high push-up position, with your hands positioned slightly wider than shoulder-width apart, then lower yourself down into a low push-up position.

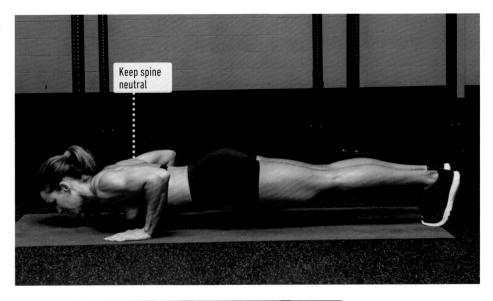

Keep spine neutral

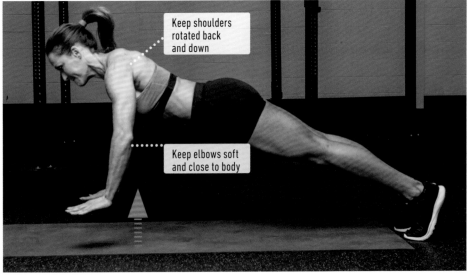

Keep shoulders rotated back and down

Keep elbows soft and close to body

[2] Explosively push your body upward with enough power to make your hands leave the ground. Land as softly as possible in the high push-up position, then quickly drop back down into the low push-up position and repeat the movement.

TARGETS **/// quads, hamstrings, calves (primary); abs, shoulders, glutes (secondary)**
EQUIPMENT **/// tape**

LINE JUMPS

Line jumps will increase your overall power and explosiveness by hitting almost every muscle in your lower body, and also getting your heart rate up. To reap the full benefit, go for maximum effort and keep the total reps to 10 or less.

TIP
Arms account for as much as 30% of a jump, so be sure to sweep the arms forward with each jump.

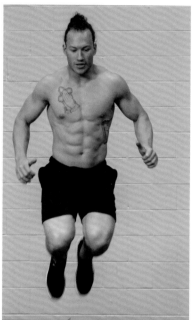

Keep weight in balls of feet

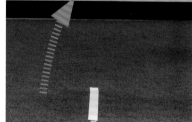

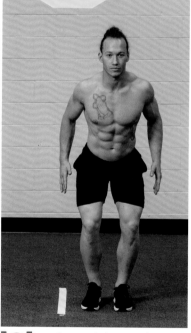

[1] Place a strip of tape on the floor. Stand with both feet shoulder-width apart and parallel to the line. Prepare for the jump by bending your knees and loading your arms behind your body.

[2] Explosively jump up and over the line by pushing from the balls of your feet and swinging your arms forward.

[3] Land on soft knees, drop back down into the starting position, and load your arms behind your body. Jump back over the line, repeating the exercise in a rapid, continuous motion.

TARGETS /// quads, calves, abs (primary); shoulders, chest (secondary)
EQUIPMENT /// bench

BENCH POPOVERS

Bench pop-overs are an excellent way to sneak some core work into your cardio routine. The benefits of this exercise include a higher calorie burn and increased jumping power.

VARIATION

Plank bunny hops (easier) From a plank position, hop up and tuck your knees up to one elbow, and then hop back to the plank position. Repeat on the opposite side.

TIP For maximum results, keep your contact time with the ground to a minimum.

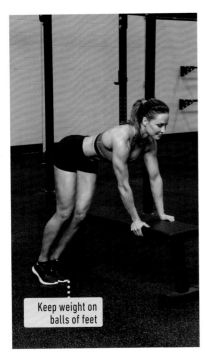

Keep weight on balls of feet

[1] Stand alongside the bench, bend forward, and grasp both sides of the bench.

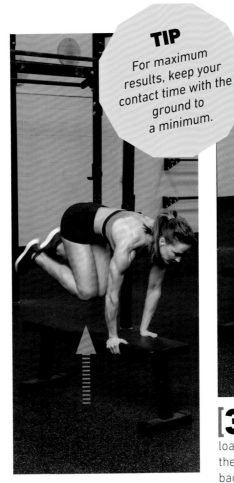

[2] With a flat back and soft elbows, bend your knees to generate power, then jump up and "pop" over to the other side of the bench. while keeping a firm grasp on the bench.

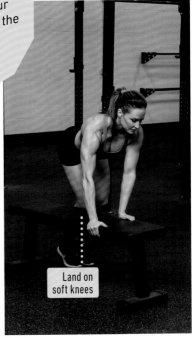

Land on soft knees

[3] Land softly on the balls of your feet, then immediately load your legs and jump back over the bench. Repeat in a rapid, back-and-forth motion.

TARGETS /// hamstrings, glutes, calves (primary); abs, shoulders (secondary)
EQUIPMENT /// none

BUTTKICKS

Buttkicks will fire up your glutes and hamstrings, and get your blood pumping! Over time, you'll improve coordination, core strength, and balance.

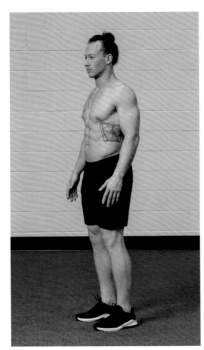

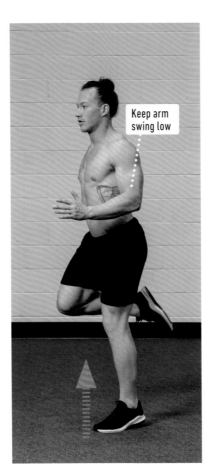

Keep arm swing low

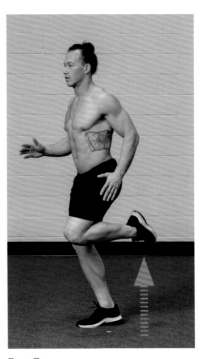

[1] Stand with your feet positioned shoulder-width apart, your upper body tall, and your arms relaxed at your sides. Shift your balance to the balls of your feet.

[2] Keeping your upper legs as perpendicular to ground as possible, kick your lower leg up and back towards your glutes, while simultaneously swinging the opposite arm up and forward, and swinging the opposing arm behind your body.

[3] Quickly bring your lower leg back down to the starting point while simultaneously kicking the opposite leg up and back and swinging the opposite arm forward. Repeat in a rapid, continuous motion.

INDEX

U–V

W

X–Y–Z